How Healthy People Eat

An Eater's Guide To Healthy Habits

By Kristen Coffield

How Healthy People Eat
An Eater's Guide To Healthy Habits

Text by Kristen Coffield
Graphic design by Becca Stewart

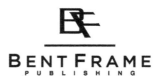

BENT FRAME
PUBLISHING

NEW YORK

Edited by Kaitlin Puccio, Esq.
NASM FNS (Fitness Nutrition Specialist)

www.bentframepublishing.com

For my children, Will, Jessie, and Virginia, who learned to love broccoli, sweet potatoes, and water in a world of Hot Pockets and Slurpees.

Table of Contents

Introduction

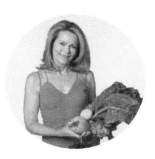

Healthy people have habits that contribute to their overall vitality and wellness. The things they do give them resilience, mental clarity, boundless energy, proper body weight, and the ability to effectively deal with stress.[1] In a nutshell, healthy habits contribute to a healthy life.

When it comes to healthy habits, eating is powerful. What we eat, how we eat, and when we eat all matter. Mastering daily food habits is a tool we can use to create culinary resilience—the ultimate wellness benefit. When we give our bodies what they need to thrive, we are rewarded with a strong immune system,[2] lower inflammation,[3] and lots of feel-good hormones.[4]

We all need to trade habits that do not serve us for habits that do. When we understand that our food practices are opportunities to fuel our health and happiness, we can be more mindful of our choices. How Healthy People Eat is a kitchen companion filled with little bites of information to motivate, inspire, and empower you to develop culinary resilience by using food as your superpower.

One morsel at a time we can change our wellness destiny. By creating better habits, we can reset our health to the factory settings with which we were born and eat in a way that supports looking, feeling, and being well. Think of this little book as the first bite to help you harness the nutritive power on the end of your fork.

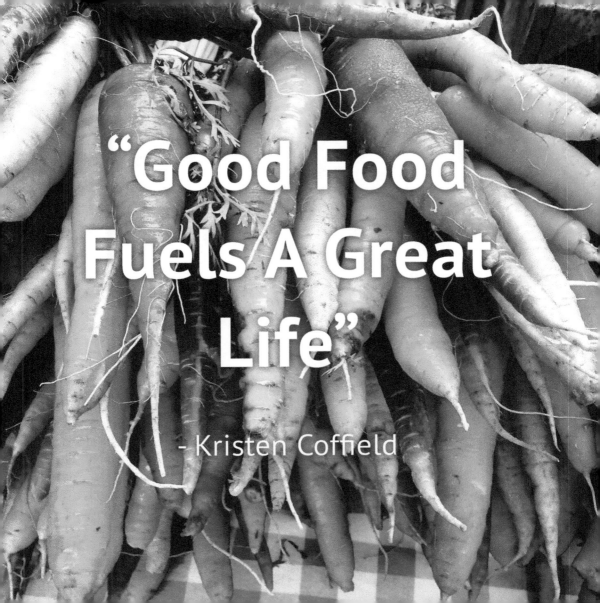

"Good Food Fuels A Great Life"

- Kristen Coffield

EAT WELL.
BE WELL.

The little things we do over and over again have a big impact on our lives.

If we want to get good at something, we first need to get started. If we want to become an expert, we need to be consistent, logging thousands of dedicated hours toward the goal we want to achieve. Our challenge here is to think of this in relation to what we eat and drink.

We will spend over thirty-two thousand hours eating in our lifetime.[5] That's ample time to become an eating expert. During those hours, we will consume millions of calories that give our bodies the energy they need to operate.[6] We need to be smart about where we get these calories, however, as many staples of the Western diet lack the nutrient diversity we need to thrive.[7] Our cells use calories to initiate important metabolic processes, extracting micro- and macro-nutrients from food that can influence everything from cell function to gene expression.[8] These processes depend on nutrients to create energy, regulate hormones, and construct many building blocks of our body chemistry.[9]

Our gut—or microbiome—calls the shots that affect our overall wellness, using what we eat and drink as chemical instructions.[10]

Eating the right things means giving our bodies the fuel they are pre-wired to use to keep us healthy. Consuming foods and beverages that the body does not recognize or know how to break down has the opposite effect. Poor consumption creates inflammation, and inflammation is no small problem.[11] Low-level chronic inflammation is linked to weight gain, diabetes, neurological decline, heart disease, cancer, and other destructive diseases[12].

When I talk about "real food," I'm talking about food as close to its natural state as possible. Real food is minimally processed and without added chemicals, sugar, salt, and modified fats. Our bodies know what to do with real food. Typically, the best food for us will also be better for the planet.[13] It will be sustainably and humanely raised and farmed without excessive chemicals.[14] We have to remember that we are what we eat <u>and</u> what our food eats.

What we eat matters. *How* we eat matters, too. Our mothers were right when they told us to slow down and chew our food because digestion begins with chewing.[15] As we chew, we activate digestive chemicals in our mouths that first break down food in preparation for nutrient absorption.[16] Eating fast, not properly chewing our food, and washing food down with liquids all interfere with this process.[17]

We can eat well to be well. We simply need to create everyday food practices that nourish and support our bodies and minds.

BUY LESS FOOD

Annually Americans throw away more than 38 million tons of food per year. The price tag attached to that is $165 billion dollars per year.

Graphic: source[18]

In 2012, the nutritional value of wasted food contained enough nutrients to feed 190 million adults every day for a year.[19] The environmental impact of this food waste is massive, too. As organic waste breaks down in landfills around the world, it creates over 4 billion tons of carbon dioxide.[20] That's more greenhouse gas than is produced by any one country, with the exception of the United States and China.[21] Global food waste is one of the biggest contributors to climate change, but it's not too late to start cultivating sustainable habits.[22] Buy less and have a plan for all the food you bring home.

EAT WELL. BE WELL.

BUY BETTER FOOD

Think of food as fuel.
Your body knows what to do
with food; it doesn't know
what to do with highly
processed products with
chemical additives.

Graphic: source[23]

We are omnivores, and we need to eat the proper fuel to function optimally.[24]
The Western Diet contains too many chemicals, too much added sugar, too
much factory-farmed protein, and too many refined carbohydrates.[25] Rather than
eating like omnivores, we are eating like carnivores who eat carbohydrates,
creating unhealthy inflammation in our bodies.[26] A plant-rich diet supports
good health.[27] Buy the best-quality food you can afford, organic when possible,
and mostly plants.

EAT ALL THE FOOD YOU BUY

Have a plan for the food you buy. Most people shop for food, rather than shopping for meals.

We all know that getting through a workweek requires stamina, focus, and restorative rest. The food we choose can support our goals by fueling us effectively. Having a meal plan for the week allows us to shop with intention, prepare nutritious snacks and meals, and save time and money. We only need four and a half days of food to get us through the busiest part of our week, and planning in advance ensures that we'll have everything we need to keep going. Make a list, stick to it, and meal prep on Sunday before the week gets busy.

EAT WELL. BE WELL.

CONSUME LESS ANIMAL PROTEIN

Eating a diet with large amounts of animal protein is linked to increased risks of heart disease, cancer, diabetes, obesity, and antibiotic resistance.

Graphic: source[28]

Industrial farming practices have made meat cheap and available.[29] The average American consumes more than 10 ounces per day of animal protein.[30] We don't have to give up meat completely, but we do need to think differently about how we consume it. Buying humanely raised meat and using it as an accompaniment instead of the main course will add flavor, fat, and protein to plant-rich dishes and help with overall portion control. There's a reason my family's plates are always 75% vegetables![31]

READ LABELS

We should only buy foods that have short lists of recognizable ingredients.

I only reach for non-GMO whole fruits, vegetables, legumes, nuts, seeds, grains, beans, fungi, and humanely-raised animal products. These deliver the most nutritional benefits, and the body knows what to do with them.[32] Artificial chemicals, preservatives and other additives are NOT food, and the body does NOT know what to do with them.[33] Avoiding processed, chemically-enhanced foods is more beneficial for the body.[34] Here's what I always say: If you can't pronounce it, your body probably can't process it.

EAT WELL. BE WELL.

BUY FOOD WITH LESS INGREDIENTS

The REAL problem is that food labels do NOT define a food as being good or bad for human consumption.

Food labels simply tell us how a food *might* fit into our daily diet and what percentage of nutrients we *might* be getting. They don't tell us if we're eating what our bodies need or whether a particular diet is even the right one to keep us healthy. As a rule, the more ingredients listed on a food label, the more processed the food is likely to be. If there are ingredients we can't identify, they are likely chemicals designed to extend shelf life, improve the way a food looks, or make the food addictively delicious.[35] Remember, ingredients like these won't help us become healthier.[36]

EAT WELL. BE WELL.

ADD FERMENTED FOODS TO YOUR DIET

Fermenting foods has been practiced for centuries as a way to extend the freshness of grains, animal products, fruits, and vegetables.

The simple, natural process of fermenting foods has many health advantages. Fermented foods are high in nutrients, digestion-enhancing enzymes, and fiber.[37] They also deliver powerful servings of beneficial bacteria that contribute to a healthy gut microbiome.[38] Make fermented foods a regular part of your meals, and have fun incorporating their unique flavors into your favorite dishes. My Fermented Salsa Fresca is a tangy twist on a classic party dip, and you can find the recipe on theculinarycure.com.

EAT WELL. BE WELL.

BE AWARE THAT NUTRITION LABELS ARE NOT 100% ACCURATE!

The FDA accepts a 20% margin of error in labeling.

Graphic: source[39]

That means the listed calories, sugars, total fat, saturated fat, cholesterol, carbohydrates, and sodium can actually be up to 20% higher than what is stated on the label![40] A product label may claim that one serving contains just 19 grams of fat, but, in reality, this serving could contain 23 grams. Despite this error, the product would still be in compliance with FDA regulations. Buy fewer foods that require a food label, and minimize the risk of being misinformed.

SWAP YOUR SWEETENER

When we eat sugar, we are feeding our bad gut bacteria, which in turn creates sugar cravings.

Graphic: source[41]

Sugar disrupts us mentally and physically; the more we consume it, the more we crave it.[42] Weaning off sugar and artificial sweeteners can be challenging, but it's worth it. A tough period of paring back on sugar is a small price to pay for a healthier future. Because sugar is linked to inflammation in the body,[43] we want to minimize added sugars and enjoy natural sugars that are found in whole fruits and vegetables. A little raw, unfiltered honey, grade-B maple syrup, or blackstrap molasses will be enough to sweeten most things. Break your sweetener habit and never look back.

EAT WELL. BE WELL.

SWITCH TO HEALTHIER SALT

Most people consume five times the amount of dietary sodium necessary for good health.

Graphic: source[44]

Elevated sodium is linked to high blood pressure and adversely affects our blood vessels, heart, kidneys, and brain.[45] The problem lies in processed salt or table salt, otherwise known as sodium chloride.[46] Sodium chloride is salt chemically stripped of its beneficial, naturally occurring nutrients and minerals.[47] I think of this white table salt and white sugar as evil co-conspirators, as both are over-processed, addictive, dangerous to our health, and used generously in processed foods.[48] The best salt for our health is Himalayan crystal salt, formed before the oceans were polluted.[49] It contains over 80 essential minerals and trace elements that benefit our health.[50] Get a little container, bring your own salt when dining out, and toss the sodium chloride lurking in your cabinets.

EAT WELL. BE WELL.

DON'T DRINK LIQUIDS WITH MEALS

Digestion begins with chewing food and activating enzymes in your mouth.

Graphic: source[51]

Some studies suggest that washing food down with liquids dilutes digestive enzymes and causes our stomachs to secrete more acids to break down food.[52] I like to make sure that I am well hydrated before sitting down for a meal, and I wait 20 minutes after a meal before consuming more liquids. If your friends look at you funny when you refuse a drink with dinner, explain how liquids negatively affect digestion, and invite them to join you on your path toward smarter eating.

EAT WELL. BE WELL.

USE FOOD AS A PRODUCTIVITY TOOL

Food is fuel.
Food powers our bodies
and minds.

Graphic: source[53]

Once we know how and what to eat, we can harness the natural power of whole, real foods. Food can and should be so much more than "empty" calories; it represents one of the most valuable tools we have in improving our overall quality of life. Using food as medicine to keep us healthy is totally possible and absolutely priceless.

EAT WELL. BE WELL.

SNACK BETTER

Plan healthy snacks.
Everyone gets caught
skipping meals, fueling on
caffeine, and turning hangry.

Our best line of defense is planning clean energy for busy days—simple snacks that can travel and work well on the fly. Bags of crunchy chickpeas, an apple or orange, cheese cubes, little bags of nuts, and hard-boiled eggs can all be in our arsenal of emergency rations. Always keep some handy, and protect yourself from bad choices brought on by hanger.

EAT WELL. BE WELL.

FEED YOUR GOOD GUT BACTERIA

You are what you eat, and you are also the gut bacteria that you feed.

Graphic: source[54]

Eating a plant-rich diet provides us with nutrients, fiber, and enzymes that nourish every cell in our bodies and support good gut health.[55] Eating a diet filled with processed carbohydrates, chemical additives, and added sugar has the exact opposite effect.[56] When we eat a highly processed diet, we feed the bad gut bacteria and create inflammation and cravings.[57] Use the tips and tricks in this book to guide your shopping cart toward foods that support your gut and immune system.

EAT LESS ADDED SUGAR

Real, processed, and fake sugars are ALL bad for us in excess.

Graphic: source[58]

With this in mind, the only sugar I endorse is the natural sugar found in whole fruits and vegetables.[59] Naturally occurring sugar in plants is always accompanied by fiber, which is known to slow the rate at which sugar is released into our bloodstream, tempering the insulin response.[60] Read labels, scan for sugar's alternative names like sucrose or syrup, and pay attention to the total amount of sugar. According to the American Heart Association, the daily recommended amount of added sugar is 9 teaspoons for men and 6 teaspoons for women, which equals just 36 grams and 24 grams, respectively.[61] Remember, like salt, sugar is also addictive.[62] Eat sweet, crave sweet—so avoid added sugars whenever possible.

EAT WELL. BE WELL.

AVOID FRANKENFOODS

Frankenfoods are created in factories and laboratories, and are chemically enhanced to taste delicious and be addictive.

Graphic: source[63]

An apple is an apple. Real food doesn't come with labels because it doesn't need them. Real foods are becoming increasingly hard to find, however; the total number of products in the average grocery store has increased by over 600% since the 1990s, reflecting a proliferation of frankenfoods chock-full of harmful chemical additives.[64] In a world where grocery store shelves are packed with shiny, new products, we have to remember that artificial chemicals are not food.[65] Artificial ingredients and sweeteners are unhealthy, and foods that do not occur in nature are merely food-like substances with little or no nutritional value.[66]

EAT WELL. BE WELL.

STOP EATING BEFORE YOU ARE FULL

Americans are some of the most overfed, nutritionally-deficient people on the planet.

Graphic: source[67]

Our dietary blunders are due in part to the fact that we're not actively listening to our bodies before, during, and after we eat. We eat in our cars, in front of screens, and when we should be sleeping. Slowing down and chewing each bite can help us understand how full we feel.[68] Before reaching for seconds—which means more calories, more stress on our digestive system, and more pounds around our waistlines—we need to give our bodies time to register fullness. Learn what 80% full feels like, because you are really 100% full.[69]

EAT WELL. BE WELL.

KEEP A FOOD JOURNAL

A record of what you eat and drink is a powerful tool.

For one week, write down everything you eat and drink (including the amount, the time, and who you were with), in addition to how much water you drink throughout the day and how much sleep you get each night. You will begin to see patterns. Shortchanging ourselves on sleep can lead us to make poor dietary choices,[70] drink more caffeine, and eat more sugar.[71] Not drinking enough water can also lead to poor food and beverage choices.[72] Use your food journal to help you improve your habits so that they can be used to benefit your health.

PRACTICE
MINDFUL EATING

Eating while walking, driving, standing in front of the refridgerator, or sitting in front of the computer are all bad habits that detract from mindful enjoyment of our food.

Set times for mindful eating, and look forward to scheduled snacks and meals throughout the day instead of indulging when bored. The "right" foods will keep us fuller longer and minimize cravings, whereas eating processed, sugary foods makes us hungry for more.[73] We can set ourselves up for success by preparing nutrient-dense foods, and we should give ourselves time to sit down, eat slowly, and savor every flavor several times a day. Not only do we deserve these moments, but hurried eating is bad for digestion and is linked to overeating and other poor food choices.[74]

EAT WELL. BE WELL.

START YOUR DAY WITH FUEL

Eat foods that contain fiber, fat, and protein to start your day.

A high-protein diet helps decrease hunger-stimulating hormones.[75] Healthy fats, from olive oil and nuts for example, fuel our brains and keep us feeling fuller longer.[76] Fiber helps to feed our good gut bacteria and benefits digestion.[77] My website, theculinarycure.com, is full of balanced breakfast recipes; check out the Mini Vegetable Frittatas or Pumpkin Spice Power Balls as a great way to start your day.

REPLACE TABLE SALT WITH MISO OR SEAWEED SALT

Miso is a fermented soy product that has numerous health benefits.

Seaweed salt is made from kelp and is an excellent natural source of iodine, which is good for our thyroid gland.[78] Miso is also beneficial for immune support and breast, bone, joint, and cardiovascular health.[79] It is high in zinc and other minerals that help the body heal and keep blood vessels and joints functioning properly.[80] I love to use miso as a health-boosting salt substitute. It works beautifully in salad dressings, sauces, and marinades. Of course, you can also use it to make miso soup!

EAT WELL. BE WELL.

DRINK MORE GREEN TEA

Green tea is one of the healthiest beverages you can drink.

Graphic: source[81]

Powerful phytonutrients called polyphenols are exclusive to the tea plant and are linked to prevention of cancer and many other diseases.[82] Cold-steep organic green tea bags overnight in your refrigerator to make refreshing iced green tea. Try a matcha latte with almond or oat milk in place of your morning coffee, but watch out for added sweetener!

USE WALNUT OIL IN SALAD DRESSINGS

Walnuts have some of the highest antioxidant and omega-3 levels of any nut.

Graphic: source[83]

Not only is walnut oil delicious in salad dressings and sprinkled on vegetables, a 35-gram serving provides as much nutritional benefit as 50 grams of whole walnuts, as long as it's fresh and uncooked.[84] Look for unrefined walnut oil as an excellent source of essential fatty acids.[85]

EAT WELL. BE WELL.

EAT 1 TABLESPOON GROUND RAW FLAXSEED

Flaxseeds have powerful benefits!

Packed with powerful antioxidants, flaxseeds can help improve digestion, balance hormones, benefit cardiovascular health, and minimize sugar cravings.[86] You can add flaxseeds to a variety of recipes, but you can also harness their health benefits by consuming them on their own, like a supplement. Ground or milled flaxseed is easier to digest than whole flaxseed, but if you prefer to buy whole flaxseed in bulk, you can grind the seeds at home with a coffee grinder or food processor.[87] Add 1 tablespoon of ground, raw flaxseed to your food or stir into 8 ounces of filtered water and drink daily.

DRINK
MORE
WATER

Water is the healthiest
beverage you can drink.

Graphic: source[88]

Get a pitcher with a filter feature, measure your water intake throughout the day, and try to drink 100 ounces before 5pm each evening. Do not drink your water all at once, but instead sip it throughout the day. Being well-hydrated is associated with healthier food and beverage choices.[89] Drinking more water also reduces the risk of heart disease and improves cognitive function.[90] Be sure to buy a BPA-free reusable water bottle and minimize single-use plastics.

EAT WELL. BE WELL.

DRINK HIBISCUS TEA

Make hibiscus tea your go-to health beverage.

Hibiscus tea is packed with nutrients, antioxidants, and anticancer properties.[91] It can help reduce high blood pressure, lower cholesterol, relieve symptoms of anxiety, improve digestion, and boost the immune system.[92] Make a pitcher of hibiscus tea using one hibiscus tea bag for every 16 ounces of water. Let steep for 12 or more hours and sip throughout the day.

EAT AND DRINK MORE PLANT-RICH FOODS

Eating a diet rich in plant foods like fruits, vegetables, nuts, seeds, and whole grains helps prevent disease.

Graphic: source[93]

Diet has become the leading cause of death in the United States.[94] It's time we understand how to become smarter consumers and chefs. Avoiding added sugars, chemicals, processed foods, large amounts of animal products, and refined carbohydrates helps minimize the risk of disease.[95] Eating this way is better for us and better for the planet.[96] Start with the simple principles in this section, and realize that healthier eating can be easy, accessible, and absolutely delicious.

EAT WELL. BE WELL.

"Big Change Starts with Small Action"

- Kristen Coffield

FOOD IS MEDICINE

"Let food be thy medicine and medicine be thy food."
– attributed to Hippocrates

The human body contains 30 trillion cells and almost 40 trillion bacteria that support our eleven major organ systems.[97] The list of nutrients required to run our bodies is extensive, including six essential nutrients that our bodies cannot make on their own: carbohydrates, fats, proteins, vitamins, minerals, and water.[98] Making things more complicated, there are over 20 thousand genes in the human body[99] that can be affected by things in our environment, including what we eat and drink.[100]

The food we eat communicates with our genes, and what we consume can actually alter our gene expression.[101] Even more interesting is the fact that "functional whole foods" contain a collective group of nutrients that work together to promote our overall well-being.[102] Unlike some functional foods that undergo fortification during processing, functional *whole* foods include plants, animals, and fungi that contain a range of nutrients in their natural form. These are the foods that have been feeding humans for millennia. They support our bodies and brains,[103] protect our health, and keep bad stuff from damaging our genes.[104]

In a nutshell, by eating a diet filled with things our bodies are pre-programmed to utilize, we can cultivate wellness and avoid disease.[105] The daily habit of eating—something we already do to survive—can become an opportunity to thrive. We just need to learn how to eat well. Fortunately, there is a simple formula to guide us in the right direction. Before you eat or drink, ask yourself:

Is It FOOD?

F Free of chemicals
O Once alive
O OK for you and the planet
D Delivers nutrients

ADZUKI BEANS

Add these to your
culinary arsenal and
detoxify your system!
Adzuki beans are full of
digestible fiber and
protein, as well as lots of
folic acid and B vitamins.

Graphic: source[106]

The real draw with adzuki beans is their high content of trace minerals.[107] They are stuffed with molybdenum, a mineral necessary for the production of sulfite oxidase, which is in turn vital to the process of liver detoxification.[108] Poor detoxification can lead to a slew of serious conditions, such as Parkinson's and Alzheimer's diseases, as well as rheumatoid arthritis and inflammatory issues.[109] Sauté a plate of adzuki beans with herbs and spices or use them to spruce up a good salad to tap into their health benefits while making delicious meals.

FOOD IS MEDICINE

ALMONDS

Fuel for the whole day in the palm of your hand! The amount of nutrition and energy held within these tiny little things is… well, nuts.

Just a 1/3-cup serving of almonds contains 280 calories, 24 grams of healthy fat, 5 grams of fiber, and 10 grams of protein.[110] Once a coveted ingredient in the bread of pharaohs,[111] almonds provide a great source of potassium, calcium, iron, zinc, magnesium, and vitamin E.[112] They contain several important antioxidant flavonoids and supply the body with crazy amounts of energy in extremely manageable servings.[113] They are most nutritious eaten raw,[114] making almonds a perfect source of power for people on plant-based, raw diets.

Graphic: source[115]

It's no wonder the Aztecs believed amaranth gave them supernatural strength and endowed them with magical power.[116] Amaranth is unique in its supply of the essential amino acids lysine and methionine.[117] Lysine in particular is almost never found in grains, making amaranth a standout option.[118] In addition to its protein value, it is significantly less allergenic than many other grains and is naturally gluten-free.[119] Recent studies also suggest that amaranth is an excellent food choice for those with cholesterol and cardiovascular issues.[120] Enjoy amaranth in bean dishes, sides, or baked goods.

BRAZIL NUTS

These Amazonian wonders are full of cancer-fighting, heart-healthy nutrients and minerals.

Graphic: source[121]
High in protein and healthy polyunsaturated fats, the Brazil nut is also full of selenium and chromium, two extremely beneficial trace minerals.[122] At the recommend levels, selenium reduces heart disease and cancer risk, while working against inflammation and allergies.[123] Chromium aids the body's production and response to insulin, thereby lowering blood sugar.[124] These two essential components make Brazil nuts a healthy, worthwhile snack, one you can keep in your car or purse for a filling pick-me-up on the go.

BUCKWHEAT

Bolster your immune system with the flavonoid richness of buckwheat!

Graphic: source[125]

Originating in Central Asia, the buckwheat seed holds many valuable nutritional properties, thanks to its supply of two superstar flavonoids: rutin and quercetin.[126] Both rutin and quercetin act as antioxidants in the body, and they are both shown to improve heart health.[127] They can also prevent blood clotting and block the development of harmful cholesterols in the body.[128] Buckwheat is yet another great fiber source, and its flavonoid-fueled, blood-sugar-balancing power delivers benefits to the entire body.[129] Consider it as an alternative to flour the next time you bake. Buckwheat pancakes, anyone?

FOOD IS MEDICINE

CAROB

Curb your chocolate addiction with the diverse and delicious carob plant.

Growing in long, slightly curved fruit pods, these sweet, brown seeds can be eaten fresh, roasted, or ground to be used like cocoa powder. Carob requires no additional sweetening and is virtually fat-free.[130] It is low in calories, high in fiber, and stuffed with vitamins A, B2, B3, B6, E, D, and C.[131] All these healthy qualities make carob a tasty and nutritious alternative to chocolate, so you can satisfy your sweet tooth in a healthier way.

CASHEWS

Don't miss out on the crunchy goodness of these protein-packed snacks!

Cashews are actually a seed.[132] They are unique in that they contain much less fat and more protein than most tree nuts.[133] Their fat content is derived from extremely beneficial oleic acid, which is a monounsaturated oil that has been shown to help protect against cancer and heart disease.[134] The cashew also supplies magnesium, potassium, copper, iron, and zinc.[135] Fuel up and keep a happy heart by adding them to your trail mix!

CHIA SEEDS

Maximize nutrients and minimize calories with the ultra-efficiency of chia seeds!

Named after the Mayan word for "strength,"[136] chia seeds pack 11 grams of fiber, 4 grams of protein, 9 grams of fat, and tons of calcium, manganese, magnesium, and phosphorus in a single ounce at only 137 calories.[137] Chia seeds are completely whole-grain, naturally gluten-free, and loaded with antioxidants.[138] Indeed, this superfood makes the hunt for valuable nutrients on an alternative diet a whole lot easier. Even if you're not dieting, consider introducing chia seeds to your regular rotation for their high fiber and protein content. Add them to your morning yogurt bowl, for example. Starting the day with chia seeds is always a good idea. Get my favorite recipe for Chia Seed Pudding at theculinarycure.com.

CHICKPEAS

With a Latin title translating to "small ram," the nutritional force that is the powerful chickpea more than lives up to its name.

Graphic: source[139]

Chickpeas are the ideal low-fat, high-protein food; their comforting texture and taste makes them a welcome addition to an array of recipes from many diverse cultures.[140] Also known as the garbanzo bean, chickpeas contain large amounts of fiber, protein, folate, manganese, copper, and zinc.[141] Chickpeas also have an abundance of molybdenum, a mineral that can detoxify sulfite.[142] Sulfite is a common preservative found in foods and wine that can cause headaches, abdominal pain, hives, and worse for those with sulfite sensitivities.[143] With the right herbs and spices, you can deliciously harness the detoxifying powers of chickpeas and make them an integral component of healthy home-cooked meals.

COCONUTS

Big, hairy health questions have a big, hairy answer! The coconut contains lauric acid, which naturally converts into an extremely beneficial compound called monolaurin.

Graphic: source[144]

Found only in coconut fat and breast milk, monolaurin fights all kinds of disease-causing organisms, such as those related to the flu, measles, and even HIV.[145] In addition to its impressive antimicrobial and antiviral properties, coconut meat is replete with health-boosting nutrients; its high manganese content, for example, promotes bone health and the metabolism of essential vitamins.[146] Add shredded, unsweetened coconut to oats or granola, and try coconut flour as a high-fiber and gluten-free alternative to white flour when baking. You can also harness the health benefits of coconut oil by using extra virgin coconut oil for all your cooking needs.

COCONUT OIL

One simple, healthy ingredient for all your cooking needs. Coconut oil is the single best oil for sautéing, baking, and stir-frying.

Despite noisy controversies surrounding coconut oil's high saturated fat content, coconut oil remains a superior, highly stable source of plant-based fat.[147] Whereas the high linoleic acid content in vegetable oils may increase the risk of cardiovascular disease,[148] coconut oil can actually reduce the risk of heart disease by increasing our "good" cholesterol levels.[149] Unlike other saturated fats, coconut oil is composed of medium-chain fatty acids, which greatly benefit liver health and energy metabolism.[150] Coconut oil's low level of polyunsaturated oil makes it an ideal fat for high-heat cooking,[151] and it's mild flavor will add a delicate richness to your favorite recipes. As you begin updating your pantry with nutritious alternatives to unhealthy ingredients, coconut oil is a good addition.

FOOD IS MEDICINE

FLAXSEEDS

Fight back against heart disease, and even cancer, with this simple but powerful seed!

Graphic: source[152]

Chock-full of alpha-linolenic acid, flaxseeds provide a litany of imperative health benefits.[153] Alpha-linolenic acid (ALA), like other omega-3 fatty acids, has shown great promise in its ability to reduce the risk of heart disease, and flaxseeds are replete with ALA.[154] Just one tablespoon of flaxseed oil contains nearly 6 times the amount of omega-3 fatty acids found in a 3-ounce serving of cooked salmon.[155] Flaxseeds also contain substantial amounts of dietary fiber and lignans, which can disrupt cancer-promoting effects of estrogen on breast tissue.[156] Additionally, studies show that the consumption of flaxseed is a great way to reduce bad cholesterol.[157] For short-term deliciousness and long-term wellness, look no further than the nutrient-rich flaxseed.

Graphic: source[158]

Hemp seeds provide all nine essential amino acids, while also containing great quantities of vitamin E, magnesium, phosphorous, potassium, niacin, riboflavin, thiamine, vitamin B6, and folate.[159] These small but massively impressive seeds include can reduce inflammation, improve skin conditions, and bolster overall heart health.[160] Their content of cannabidiol (CBD) also suggests that they can be helpful in managing neurological conditions such as Alzheimer's and Parkinson's.[161] There are many culinary uses of the hemp seed—they make a great addition to pasta, pudding, and smoothies!

HIMALAYAN PINK SEA SALT

The same salty satisfaction plus 84 extra nutrients!

Graphic: source[162]

Cultivated from the Khewra Salt Mine, located close to the Himalayas in Pakistan, this pink-colored salt is minimally processed, making it a much more natural alternative to your average table salt.[163] The Khewra Mine's ancient properties and the natural means by which the salt is cultivated gives Himalayan pink sea salt a far superior supply of minerals.[164] This supply includes calcium, potassium, magnesium, molybdenum, iron, and sodium; it can contain up to 84 combined minerals and elements.[165] Though it's important to monitor overall sodium intake, Himalayan salt offers much greater nutritional value than regular table salt.

KELP GRANULES AND FLAKES

This special seaweed provides extraordinary supplies of iodine, as well as other important minerals, vitamins, and antioxidants.

Graphic: source[166]

Kelp granules and flakes have been proven to fight dangerous cancer cells, specifically those responsible for breast and colon cancers.[167] Iodine-rich foods like kelp have also been shown to nurture infant brain development.[168] This seaweed isn't just for developing brains, though; it helps us maintain healthy skin, hair, and eyes.[169] On top of all these incredible benefits, kelp provides essential amino acids, omega-3 fats, and digestible fiber.[170] Make your next salad even healthier with this simple addition.

LENTILS

Keep your stomach full
and your blood sugar
in check with the
fiber-iffic power of the
lentil.

Supplementing diets since 8,000 B.C., lentils remain a leading source of protein, folate, and cholesterol-lowering fiber.[171] Their high fiber content prevents blood sugar from spiking after a meal, making lentils a great food for people with blood sugar disorders.[172] Additionally, researchers found a significant decrease in breast cancer frequency among women with high dietary intakes of lentils and beans.[173] For such a small food, lentils have enormous nutritional value and many diverse uses. Add them to your next homemade soup, salad, or pilaf.

MILLET

Eliminate your wheat problems with millet magic! This grain surpasses wheat, corn, and rice in protein content.

Graphic: source[174]

In addition to packing an impressive protein punch, millet also provides an excellent source of phosphorous, magnesium, thiamine, riboflavin, niacin, folate, and vitamin B6.[175] Its hypoallergenic and gluten-free properties make it a perfect, healthier alternative to wheat.[176] Millet is a whole grain through and through, meaning that it offers valuable protection against diabetes, cancer, and heart problems thanks to its high fiber content.[177] Sub it in for wheat in your baking recipes, or pair it with morning fruit.

MISO

So much more than a sushi appetizer, miso is known to be effective in preventing cancer—specifically, breast cancer.

Miso is filled with protein and digestible fiber, along with an abundance of helpful minerals like iron, copper, zinc, phosphorous, and manganese.[179] While cooking it into a soup is its most popular use, you can also incorporate miso into marinades for fish and meat. Like other fermented foods, miso contains gut-friendly good bacteria, but high-heat cooking can kill these special cultures.[180] Gently add unpasteurized miso at the end of a recipe and use it in place of salt in dressings and sauces to harness its probiotic benefits. Keep your meals interesting by letting your guests find a familiar taste in a new place!

NUTRITIONAL YEAST

Take advantage of the mineral richness and protein goodness of this healthy yeast!

Nutritional yeast is grown to be used in food, and the yeast cells within it are killed during its cultivation process.[181] It is a complete protein, containing every essential amino acid, as well as tons of B vitamins, antioxidants, and healthy minerals like zinc, selenium, manganese, and molybdenum.[182] Vitamin B12 in particular keeps the nervous system working as it should, but it's near impossible to find in a plant-based diet.[183] Nutritional yeast contains an abundance of B12, making it a good option for vegans.[184] Known for its naturally cheesy flavor, nutritional yeast can also serve as a yummy, vegan substitute for dairy products.

OATS

Experience the mineral magic of the hearty oat! These great little breakfast additions have tons of manganese, selenium, phosphorus, magnesium, and calcium.

Graphic: source[185]

The payoff for including oats in our diet is enormous. High in vitamin B1 and dietary fiber and packed with healthy fats,[186] oats are excellent for supporting healthy cholesterol levels.[187] Incorporate them into your next baking experiment—they make for delicious muffins and breads! Opt for steel-cut oats when you need a nutrient-dense breakfast, and enjoy them alongside your favorite fresh fruits and nuts.

OLIVE OIL

Cut down on saturated fat with this essential cooking tool. Olive oil is an ideal alternative to fattier butter or lard.

Graphic: source[188]

Olive oil is rich in healthy fats, making it beneficial for cardiovascular health.[189] It also has strong anti-inflammatory qualities and contains healthy antioxidants.[190] This multifaceted oil has been proven effective against conditions such as rheumatoid arthritis and type 2 diabetes, and studies show that it may even reduce the risk of cancer.[191] Let organic extra-virgin olive oil work its wonders in your favorite recipes.

PINE NUTS

The European pine nut contains more protein than any other nut or seed.

Graphic: source[192]

Both the European pine nut and its American cousin contain hefty supplies of iron, manganese, copper, zinc, magnesium, potassium, and vitamins B1, B2, E, and K.[193] These minerals and vitamins, particularly in food form, help bolster your blood flow and keep your heartbeat in check, culminating in a powerful resistance against heart disease.[194] This, combined with the pine nut's high protein content, makes pine nuts the perfect workout snack for long-term energy, cardiovascular regulation, and body mass.

PISTACHIO NUTS

The road to a healthy heart is paved with pistachios! Studies suggest that adding pistachios to our diet improves blood cholesterol levels.

Graphic: source[195]

Pistachios are a source of magnesium and potassium,[196] and studies show that adding these nuts to your diet can protect your body from blood pressure abnormalities.[197] These tasty nuts also contain anti-inflammatory compounds.[198] The regular consumption of pistachios is a great way to be kind to your cardiovascular system. Make them a go-to snack!

PUMPKIN SEEDS

With high levels of
essential fatty acids, zinc,
and phytosterols,
pumpkin seeds have
been proven to maintain
prostate health.

Graphic: source[199]

Pumpkin seeds are also a great source of vitamins A, B1, B2, and B3, iron, calcium, magnesium, protein, and monounsaturated healthy fats.[200] Gently toast them for a fresh snack after your next jack-o-lantern carving session and take advantage of their many benefits.

QUINOA

Support your body with quinoa's extraordinary protein punch. The least allergenic grain known, quinoa contains every essential amino acid.

Graphic: source[201]

In addition to almost a dozen key vitamins and nutrients, quinoa delivers an incredible amount of high-quality protein.[202] This, paired with the fact that quinoa is also gluten-free, makes it the perfect choice for vegans and gluten-free consumers. Next time you make pasta, try switching to quinoa noodles, or match it with fresh fruit and berries for an early morning treat!

FOOD IS MEDICINE

SPELT

Make your favorite baked goods healthier with this great alternative whole grain. Spelt is unusually high in fiber and minerals compared to other grains in its grain family.

Graphic: source[203]

Spelt contains many rare and healthy complex carbohydrates.[204] In fact, it is the only grain containing mucopolysaccharides, which stimulate the immune system, lower cholesterol, and play a vital role in blood clotting.[205] Mucopolysaccharides alone give spelt loads more nutritional value than plain old wheat! Try experimenting with spelt in baked goods and side dishes.

SPIRULINA

Spirulina is a blue-green algae packed with protein and vitamins and is considered to be one of the most nutrient-dense foods on the planet.

Graphic: source[206]

The complete, high-quality protein in spirulina is comparable to the protein content in eggs, gram per gram.[207] It is one of the best plant-based sources of highly absorbable and easy-to-digest iron, and it contains 26 times more calcium than milk.[208] Spirulina is a powerful antioxidant; it can balance blood sugar, boost fat-burning during exercise, and help the body detox by binding with heavy metals.[209] Spirulina belongs in everyone's wellness arsenal.

SUNFLOWER SEEDS

This hearty snack will keep you healthy and feeling full.

Just a third of a cup of these delightful seeds gives you 24 grams of healthy fat and 11 grams of protein.[210] In addition, you get abundant servings of vitamin E, magnesium, selenium, phosphorus, copper, iron, folate, fiber, and vitamins B1, B5, and B6.[211] Folic acid in its natural form, folate, has been shown to reduce the risk of cardiovascular disease and stroke,[212] and studies suggest that selenium supplements may help the human body combat cancer, inflammation, and asthma.[213] I love adding sunflower seeds to salads and sides like my Broccoli and Asian Pear Slaw for an extra, nutritious crunch.

TAHINI

Spice up your meals and bolster your immune system with this delicious side!

Tahini is a paste made from ground sesame seeds, which means it is packed with phosphorus, magnesium, potassium, iron, and many other healthy minerals.[214] It is also rich in vitamins, including vitamins E, B1, B2, B3, B6, and B9, which all benefit cell metabolism and immune strength.[215] The biggest draw of tahini, aside from its delicious taste, is its high calcium content, which helps your body maintain bone health and muscle tone.[216] This versatile sesame paste is also high in protein and healthy unsaturated fat.[217] Consider adding it to your next dish—sweet or savory!

WALNUTS

Mankind's oldest tree-food has more to it than first meets the eye. The walnut dates back to 7,000 B.C.

Graphic: source[218]

A staple of Roman and Mediterranean diets, the walnut has a rich history.[219] Vitamin B6, copper, magnesium, phosphorus, and omega-3 acids can all be found in great quantities in this ancient nut.[220] In fact, the walnut is one of the best sources of alpha-linolenic acid, second only to the chia seed.[221] As if all that weren't enough, walnuts are also rich in protein and dietary fiber and have been shown to lower bad cholesterol and improve brain function.[222] The list of health benefits goes on and on! Toast them, snack on them, toss them in a salad, or use them to make pesto. With the walnut, you simply can't go wrong.

WASABI

Refresh your taste buds
and your body's health
with this wonderful spice!

Isothiocyanates, nutrients found in large supply within the wasabi plant, have been shown to have significant cancer-preventing properties, especially against leukemia and stomach cancer.[223] Wasabi also kills harmful bacteria found in food, such as *E. coli*,[224] and can protect your heart and respiratory system.[225] Additionally, wasabi has been proven effective in treating arthritis.[226] It's delicious, and its nutritional benefits are astronomical! Find it at your local sushi restaurant or pick it up in plant form at your health food store.

"Culinary Resilience Is A 21st Century Survival Skill"

~ Kristen Coffield

CULINARY PHARMACY

Herbs and spices have been used throughout history to treat illness.[227] The term "herb" refers to plants that do not have woody stems, though it can also be used to describe any plant with medicinal properties.[228] Spices are an aromatic plant product, and most spices are the dried bark and seeds of plants.[229] Both herbs and spices are used to flavor food, and both contain powerful compounds that can benefit our health.[230]

If used correctly, herbs and spices can protect our bodies from chronic inflammation and can be used to treat, cure, and even prevent some diseases.[231] Herbs and spices are loaded with flavor compounds, many of which are a source of beneficial antioxidants.[232] By incorporating more herbs and spices into our diet, especially those containing stress-fighting adaptogens, we can support our immune system, balance our adrenals, and stimulate liver function.[233]

In 2018, the World Health Organization estimated that nearly 90% of the World's population uses herbal treatments and other alternative medicines for their healthcare needs.[234] Though herbal medicine appears to be trending in industrialized nations like the United States,[235] many people in America still know very little about the power of plants and are unaware that many of our modern medicines originated from herbs and spices. Aspirin originated from willow bark, morphine and codeine are extracted from the poppy plant, and many other pharmaceutical drugs are derived from plant compounds.[236]

We can spice up our food and boost our health with a simple collection of flavor-boosting ingredients. Snip fresh herbs into soups and salads and onto vegetables. Generously sprinkle spices into your cooking to dial up wellness benefits and flavor. Be sure to always choose organically grown to avoid herbs and spices that have been irradiated.

A healthy future belongs to those who understand the benefits of safe, complementary, and alternative medicine. Use your culinary pharmacy of herbs and spices to harness the delicious healing power of food.

ANISE

Anise has a broad range of health benefits. It is a rich source of cancer-preventing coumarin compounds, provides intestinal support, and helps to relieve coughs.

Graphic: source[237]

Anise seed is a relative of carrots, celery, and the super-herb parsley. It possesses antifungal and antimicrobial properties, and can help protect against stomach ulcers, reduce symptoms of menopause, and regulate blood sugar.[238] Recent studies also suggest that anise seed can boost your mood and lessen the symptoms of depression.[239] Anise has a licorice-like taste and can be added to baked goods or sipped in a soothing tea.

BAY LEAVES

Bay leaves are antimicrobial, antifungal, anti-inflammatory, and protect the body from free radical damage.

Graphic: source[240]
Bay leaf is believed to help manage diabetes, support proper functioning of the heart and respiratory system, and work as a natural diuretic, flushing toxins out of the body.[241] Bay leaves have been used in a wide variety of topical skin and hair treatments, and its stress- and anxiety-reducing compounds are often featured in aromatherapy.[242] Add dried bay leaves when making stocks and stews for flavor and health benefits.

BLACK PEPPER

Freshly ground black pepper enhances the bioavailability and nutrient absorption of your food.

Graphic: source[243]

When combined with turmeric in supplement form, black pepper boosts the bioavailability of curcumin, and the two spices together can fight cancer, inflammation, and oxidation.[244] On its own, black pepper possesses antioxidant and tumor-inhibiting properties, and it helps the body maintain liver health, reduce inflammation, and promote good digestion.[245] Keep fresh organic black peppercorns in a grinder on the table and use generously. Tame added sodium in your diet by swapping salt for black pepper whenever possible.

CARDAMOM

Cardamom is a staple of traditional Chinese and Ayurvedic medicines and is valued for its anti-inflammatory and stimulant properties.

Graphic: source[246]

Cardamom is revered as the "Queen of Spices" and is known for its rich aroma and sweet and savory flavor profile.[247] Cardamom is loaded with vitamins and minerals and has been used for centuries in the treatment of digestive, cardiovascular, and circulatory disorders.[248] Cardamom also contains powerful antioxidants shown to be effective in the treatment of certain cancers.[249] This spice supports metabolism, protects our DNA, and fights systemic inflammation.[250]

Graphic: source[251]

Cayenne pepper stimulates the circulatory system,[252] kick-starts the digestive system, and helps regulate blood sugar.[253] It also boosts metabolism by supporting enzyme production essential for digestion, helping to flush harmful bacteria and toxins from the body.[254] Adding a pinch of cayenne pepper to warm lemon water in the morning is a great way to rehydrate and start your day.

CINNAMON

One of the most potent antioxidants on the planet, cinnamon has a long history in both Western and Eastern cultures as a powerful medicine.

Graphic: source[255]

Cinnamon has potent wellness properties that may protect the body from inflammation,[256] arthritis,[257] asthma,[258] cancer,[259] cardiovascular problems,[260] dyspepsia, and muscle spasms.[261] Cinnamon also helps to control blood sugar by activating the insulin receptors in our cells, making it easier for them to use blood sugar for energy.[262] I like to add cinnamon to my tea, sprinkle it onto fruit, add it to smoothies, or use it to make things taste sweeter without adding sugar.

CLOVES

Cloves are an antioxidant-packed spice containing manganese, which supports the body's metabolism of fats and carbohydrates.

Graphic: source[263]

Cloves provide as many antioxidants as blueberries and promote good oral health.[264] Though clove oil has been shown to have anticancer properties in vitro, researchers warn that excess consumption may have negative effects on our health.[265] Skip the clove oil in favor of incorporating powdered cloves into healthy baked goods instead.

CORIANDER

Coriander is antimicrobial and anti-inflammatory, promotes proper digestion, reduces blood pressure, supports the reproductive system, and lowers blood sugar.

Graphic: source[266]

Coriander is the seed of the cilantro plant. A central spice in Ayurvedic medicine,[267] coriander is used to treat high cholesterol, anemia, and eye and skin infections.[268] If you can't stand the taste of cilantro—which is a powerhouse of goodness—try incorporating coriander into your diet instead. During the summer, I love featuring coriander's unique flavor in my homemade pickled watermelon rind. Visit theculinarycure.com for my recipe, inspired by my grandmother's.

CUMIN

Compounds in cumin help neutralize carcinogens, power up antioxidants, and dial down inflammation!

Cumin has been used throughout history and across the globe to help with digestion.[270] The Sanskrit word for cumin seed, jeeraka, actually means "that which digests."[271] Cumin is frequently used in Ayurvedic medicine as a potent antiviral.[272] It is also believed to effectively treat heart disease, inflammation, insomnia, poor digestion, and weakened immune system.[273] Cumin seeds contain calcium and iron and support the absorption and assimilation of nutrients.[274]

DILL

Dill weed is an overall mood and wellness booster. Dill is anti-inflammatory and antimicrobial, and helps alleviate the symptoms of PMS, insomnia, and depression.

Graphic: source[275]

An ancient Mediterranean herb, dill once meant "to soothe."[276] In addition to its calming effects, dill also protects against free radicals and contains beneficial amounts of calcium, manganese, and iron.[277] Use dill to add flavor to soups, salads, sauces, and other recipes. My baked Alaskan cod with tomatoes and dill and simple creamy vinaigrette harness the power of this delicate herb to promote bone health, manage insulin levels, and keep you happy and healthy.[278]

GARLIC

Garlic is antibacterial, anti-inflammatory, and antimicrobial, and has many cardiovascular benefits.

Graphic: source[279]

I cannot say enough good things about the health benefits of garlic! This superfood is one of the most potent aromatics on the planet and has been used to flavor food for millennia.[280] Garlic has been shown to help lower blood pressure, reduce the risk of heart disease, stabilize blood sugar, and benefit cholesterol.[281] It can also be used to treat colds and infections.[282] After slicing or chopping fresh garlic, let it rest for 10 minutes to allow for the formation of allicin.[283] Allicin is a natural byproduct of alliinase, an enzyme activated by chopping or crushing garlic cloves, that possesses powerful anticancer properties.[284] Once the allicin is formed, you can cook garlic without compromising its healthy compounds.

GINGER

Ginger has powerful anti-inflammatory properties and has been used for thousands of years to treat mild to severe digestive issues.

Graphic: source[285]

Ginger is also used to treat pain associated with arthritis and joint aches.[286] Studies demonstrate ginger's impressive antiviral, antifungal, antiparasitic, and antimicrobial powers, and its strong antioxidant properties have been shown to fight free radicals.[287] Ginger can be used in savory and sweet recipes, like my easy weeknight Asian Pesto or Spiked Lemonade with Ginger Mint Cubes (recipes at theculinarycure.com). Ginger is delicious simmered with vegetables, tossed in a stir fry, or added to smoothies, and leftover ginger root can be used to flavor water, ice cubes, and tea.

HOLY BASIL

Holy basil (aka tulsi) is considered an adaptogen because of its ability to reduce stress.

Graphic: source[288]

Holy basil has been long used as a homeopathic remedy to treat anxiety, adrenal fatigue, hypothyroidism, and unstable blood sugar levels.[289] Widely used for its therapeutic benefits, holy basil is used to protect organs and tissues from environmental toxins such as heavy metals, external stress, and restricted blood flow.[290] It's also a rich source of vitamin K, which is essential for blood clotting and bone formation, especially in postmenopausal women.[291]

HORSERADISH

Horseradish improves digestion, helps maintain a healthy gallbladder, and contains potent antibacterial ingredients that protect us from foodborne illnesses.

Graphic: source[292]

Horseradish is loaded with antioxidants, is antimicrobial and antibacterial, and has anticancer properties.[293] Horseradish root reduces inflammation and has been used to treat respiratory illnesses and UTIs.[294] Add horseradish to salad dressings and dips for heart and health benefits. Try my Bloody Mary Salsa from theculinarycure.com for a classic party snack with an extra kick!

LEEKS

Leeks provide many of the same benefits of onions and garlic. They are antibacterial, antimicrobial, anti-inflammatory, and support bone health.

Graphic: source [295]

The vitamin A content in leeks acts as an antioxidant and protects the body from environmental pollution and free radicals.[296] Leeks also contain folate,[297] an essential vitamin for pregnant women and women who may one day become pregnant.[298] Leeks have a deliciously subtle flavor and can be used to replace onions in recipes or prepared as a braised vegetable side dish.

LEMONGRASS

Lemongrass is a powerful mood-boosting aromatic that can help reduce fatigue and anxiety.

Graphic: source[299]

The volatile oils in lemongrass are antibacterial and are believed to aid in controlling the spread of *E. coli* bacteria, responsible for many food-borne ailments.[300] Lemongrass adds a pleasant citrus flavor and aromatherapeutic quality to soups, stocks, and broths. It can be found in most Asian markets.

MINT

Mint has a multitude of health benefits. It has antimicrobial, anticancer, and anti-inflammatory properties and can act as both a breath freshener and appetite suppressant.

Graphic: source[301]

Mint has been used for centuries as a medicine and all-around wellness booster.[302] Mint contains essential vitamins and minerals and is known to support overall cognitive function.[303] It also contains vitamin A and the ever-important manganese,[304] which supports bone health and improves metabolism.[305] I love adding chopped mint to salads or a few sprigs to desserts, and mint plays a starring role in my homemade pesto.

Graphic: source[306]

Sinigrin is a phenolic compound that is released when mustard seed is ground; it is what gives mustard its spice, but it also has potent medicinal benefits.[307] Mustard was historically used to treat respiratory conditions, and some people still use the mustard seed's powerful aromatic properties to overcome chest congestion and coughs.[308] Mustard seeds grow into mustard greens, which are powerful free-radical-fighting, detoxifying, and nutritious cruciferous vegetables.[309] When shopping for the condiment, make sure to buy organic stone ground mustard with no added nasties. Fun fact: The mustard seed is a member of the Brassica family, which is related to broccoli and cabbage.[310]

Graphic: source[311]

No wonder nutmeg has long been considered beneficial for overall health and wellness! It's best to consume nutmeg in moderation, however, as some of its chemical constituents are associated with hallucinogenic effects.[312] A dash of nutmeg is delicious when added to cooked fruits, and it can also take classic cocktails to the next level. I feature nutmeg in my Cranberry Margaritas and Green Tea & Ginger Toddies. You can find recipes for these new twists on old favorites on my website, theculinarycure.com.

ONIONS

They have anticancer, antimicrobial and anti-inflammatory properties, and are loaded with flavonoids and polyphenols.

Graphic: source[313]

The powerful antioxidants found in onions have cancer-preventing properties and have been shown to increase bone density, all while fighting dangerous common microbes such as staph, strep, Candida, and *E. coli*.[314] Onions are also a rich source of prebiotics, which help to nourish a healthy gut.[315] When it comes to onions, buying organic is always the way to go; studies show that antioxidant levels are significantly higher in organically grown onions.[316] ***Pro tip:*** If raw onion gives you indigestion, try rinsing or blanching onions before use.

OREGANO

This powerhouse herb fights inflammation and infection.

Graphic: source[317]

Studies suggest that the potent antioxidants in oregano can reduce inflammation and improve cardiovascular health.[318] Powerful plant compounds in oregano, including oleanolic acid and ursolic acid, can reduce cholesterol levels and prevent the build-up of arterial plaque.[319] Oregano also has many properties that provide antimicrobial, antifungal and antiviral benefits.[320] Research suggests that oregano oil, extracted from the herb, may one day be a substitute for antibiotics.[321] Hippocrates himself believed in the antibacterial qualities of oregano and used it as an antiseptic.[322] Add oregano generously to your meals, soups, and sauces.

PARSLEY

Superfood parsley supports cardiovascular health and has anticancer and anti-inflammatory properties.

Graphic: source[323]

Parsley has so many benefits it's hard to just name a few. Rich in nutrients, including chlorophyll and carotenes, parsley is a good source of vitamins, folate, and iron.[324] Its roots are a source of the antioxidant glutathione, which deactivates cancer-causing cells and protects our eyes from age-related eye disorders.[325] Parsley is also loaded with vitamins A, C, E, and K, and nutrients such as magnesium and phosphorous,[326] which are necessary for metabolism.[327] Parsley supports digestion, keeps the kidneys clean, flushes the system, increases collagen production, and boosts overall immunity.[328] Add it to everything from smoothies and sauces to soups and salads, or try it with lemon as an herbal infusion.

ROSEMARY

Rosemary contains powerful antioxidants, anti-inflammatories, and flavonoids.

Graphic: source[329]

Rosemary helps to stimulate the immune, circulatory, and digestive systems.[330] By increasing blood flow to the brain and head, rosemary has also been shown to enhance concentration.[331] It contains carnosic acid, which is known to prevent degenerative neurological conditions by protecting the brain against free radicals.[332] The antioxidants in this superb herb support good eyesight and detoxify the liver.[333] If that's not enough, rosemary also promotes digestion by regulating contractions in the gut, providing relief from cramps and other gastrointestinal discomfort.[334] ***Pro tip:*** Wash and de-stem rosemary and freeze for later use.

SAFFRON

Saffron improves cardiovascular health, helps maintain a healthy weight by creating feelings of fullness, and protects the kidneys, eyes, heart, and brain.

Graphic: source: [335]

Saffron is fragrant and delicious, but this beautiful spice comes at a high price. It takes 75,000 crocus blossoms to produce just one pound of saffron, which is why it's so expensive.[336] Saffron is a common ingredient in Middle Eastern and Indian cooking, so look for it when dining out. When using it at home, add it to healthy home-cooked soups, stews, and grains. Indicating its wealth of health benefits, saffron adds a golden color to foods.

Graphic: source[337]

Sage is also believed to alleviate degenerative diseases such as Alzheimer's and dementia, improving both cognition and overall mood.[338] The sage leaf is thought to help balance cholesterol and support a healthy weight, and studies suggest that sage may improve insulin sensitivity.[339] One of my favorite ways to use sage is in smooth vegetable soups, which can be used like grab-and-go warm smoothies. Soups are a great way to eat more vegetables; try my Super Soup master recipe on theculinarycure.com.

SEA VEGETABLES

Sea vegetables, commonly known as a seaweed, contain a vast range of minerals.

Graphic: source[340]

No other food on earth contains as broad a range of minerals as sea vegetables.[341] In fact, minerals sourced from sea vegetables are virtually the same as those found in human blood.[342] Sea vegetables supply us with cancer-fighting lignans, as well as inflammation-reducing fucans.[343] Harness the health benefits of sea vegetables while cooking by replacing salt with seaweed.

SESAME SEEDS

The sesame seed is small but mighty. Densely packed with nutrients, sesame seeds are a great source of protein, lignans, fiber, monounsaturated fats, vitamins, minerals, and calcium.

Graphic: source[344]

The fat in sesame seeds consists of 82 percent unsaturated fatty acids.[345] Their amino acid profile matches other popular vegetarian sources of protein, including soybeans and legumes, and their calcium content far exceeds milk's.[346] The lignans in sesame seeds have potent antioxidant benefits that have been shown to lower total blood cholesterol levels.[347] Try adding raw or lightly toasted sesame seeds to salads and side dishes, tossing some in your smoothies, or sprinkling them on your avocado toast.

TARRAGON

Tarragon fights free radicals, acts as a natural numbing agent, and contains large amounts of active, volatile oils known for their antimicrobial and antibacterial properties.

Graphic: source[348]

This antioxidant-packed herb also benefits cardiovascular health, soothes agitated nerves, and promotes restful sleep.[349] Tarragon has a distinctive licorice taste and can be used to flavor everything from chicken salad to fish and eggs. I always prefer homemade salad dressings, and I use tarragon to take my simple creamy vinaigrette to the next level. Visit my website, theculinarycure.com, and add this easy recipe to your weeknight arsenal.

THYME

Thyme is a natural antibacterial and antifungal. It contains kaempferol, a flavonoid with promising benefits for reducing the risk of cardiovascular disease and certain types of cancer.

Graphic: source[350]

Thyme is loaded with active ingredients like thymol, a natural antiseptic used to treat coughs and cold symptoms, and carvacrol, which wards of harmful microbes and bacteria.[351] Carvacrol has also been shown to improve dopamine and serotonin levels, and thyme is now considered to be an important mood-boosting herb.[352] Historically, thyme was used to protect against food-borne illness, and the Romans consumed thyme to treat the effects of poison.[353] Thyme is a central flavor in my classic Herbs-de-Provence rub, which brings a sense of Southern France to main dishes featuring meat and fish.

CULINARY PHARMACY

TURMERIC

Not only is turmeric used to give curry its beautiful golden color, it also has potent anti-inflammatory and anticancer properties.

Graphic: source[354]

Turmeric is a relative of ginger that is frequently used in Ayurvedic medicine, an alternative medicine rooted in ancient India.[355] The potential healing properties and health benefits of curcumin, the active ingredient in turmeric, have garnered lots of attention in recent years.[356] Curcumin has been shown to fight cancer by killing existing cancer cells and preventing further reproduction.[357] Studies also suggest that curcumin consumption minimizes skin irritation from cancer radiation treatments[358] and reduces the risk of heart attack after coronary artery bypass surgery.[359] Turmeric is an important spice to keep on hand for regular use.

Acknowledgments

I want to thank everyone who helped me to write this kitchen companion. Becca Stewart, a fearless graphic designer, who made so many valuable contributions to this book and makes everything I do look amazing. Thank you! Eleanor Dunnigan who undertook the tedious task of researching all the footnotes and sources. She not only saved me from myself, she did it with enthusiasm and good humor. My husband, partner in crime, and editor. His excellent command of the English language and love of the semicolon made my text readable. Most importantly, loving thanks to my children who ate a plant-packed diet and were good sports about the tofu.

Disclosure:

The information in this book is based on my research and personal experience. While my sources are evidence-based and in-tune with current findings, this bite-sized book is only a quick glance into the wide, complex world of healthy eating. Every body behaves differently, and your experience with the practices and ingredients introduced this book may not look like mine. This book is intended to help you start your own wellness journey. This book is *not* intended as a substitute for consulting with your physician or health-care provider. Treating and diagnosing illness should be done under the direction of a healthcare professional.

About Kristen

Kristen Coffield is the founder and owner of The Culinary Cure™, an education website dedicated to helping people use the power of food to change their lives.

She is a passionate advocate for food as medicine. Kristen turned what was on the end of her fork into a superpower to fuel her best life, and she wants to see others do the same.

Kristen is a regular contributor on Good Morning Washington, ABC7, and Fox5, where she inspires and motivates viewers to take charge of their health with easy, plant-based recipes and nutrition and wellness tips.

Her writing has been featured in DC Refined, Great Day Washington, *Washingtonian*, and in multiple other publications. She is regularly a featured speaker and wants to inspire you to use food to "live like you mean it!"

You can get more of the good stuff by visiting Kristen at theculinarycure.com; where you can sign up for her next Master Class and download your FREE guide The Culinary Cure™ Rx: Healthy Habits 101

For daily inspiration, follow @kristencoffield on Instagram.

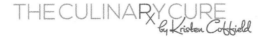

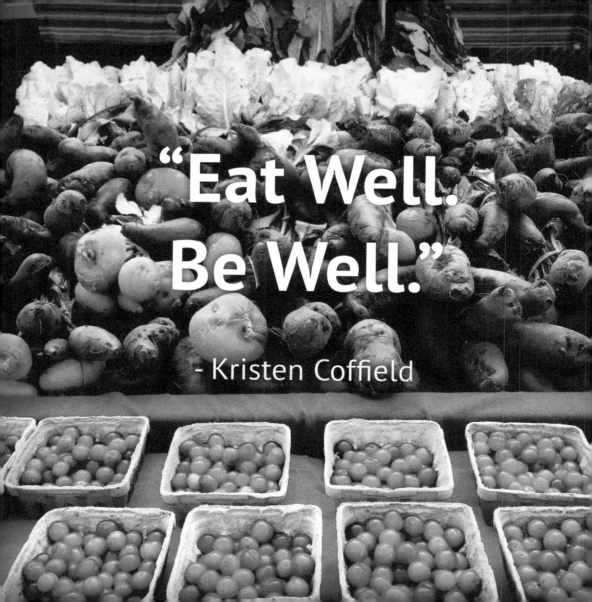

Sources

INTRODUCTION

1 Smith, Melinda, et al. "Building Better Mental Health." HelpGuide, HelpGuideOrg International, 26 Nov. 2019.

2 "How to Boost Your Immune System." Harvard Health, Harvard University, 16 July 2018.

3 "Foods That Fight Inflammation." Harvard Health, Harvard University, 7 Nov. 2018.

4 Raypole, Crystal. "Happy Hormones: What They Are and How to Boost Them." Healthline, Healthline Media, 30 Sept. 2019.

EAT WELL. BE WELL.

5 "How much time do Americans spend eating?" The Free Library. 2008 Frozen Food Digest, Inc. 24 Jan. 2020.; "Life Expectancy at Birth, Total (Years) - United States." The World Bank, The World Bank, 2019.

6 "Can You Boost Your Metabolism?" Mayo Clinic, Mayo Foundation for Medical Education and Research, 30 Aug. 2017.

7 Chen, Yiheng, et al. "Importance of Nutrients and Nutrient Metabolism on Human Health." The Yale Journal of Biology and Medicine, 91 (2), PubMed Central, 28 Jun. 2018.

8 Chen, Yiheng, et al. "Importance of Nutrients and Nutrient Metabolism on Human Health." 2018.

9 Chen, Yiheng, et al., 2018.

10 Naidoo, Uma. "Gut Feelings: How Food Affects Your Mood." Harvard Medical School, Harvard Health Publishing, 27 Mar. 2019; Corliss, Julie. "Gut Reaction: How Bacteria in Your Belly May Affect Your Heart." Harvard Medical School, Harvard Health Publishing, 8 Jul. 2016; Chen, et al. "Importance of Nutrients..." 2018.

11 Naidoo, Uma. "Gut Feelings: How Food Affects Your Mood." Harvard Health Publishing, 2019.

12 Lopez-Candales, Angel, et al. "Linking Chronic Inflammation with Cardiovascular Disease: From Normal Aging to the Metabolic Syndrome." Journal of Nature and Science, U.S. National Library of Medicine, Apr. 2017.

13 "Plate and the Planet." The Nutrition Source, Harvard T. H. Chan School of Public Health, 28 Oct. 2019.

14 "Food Sustainability." Alliance of Nurses for Healthy Environments, Alliance of Nurses for Healthy Environments, 2017.

15 Darcey, Melissa. "How Your Body Extracts Nutrients from Food, Part 2." Pathway Genomics, Pathway Genomics, 3 Apr. 2018.

16 Grodner, Michele, et al. Nutritional Foundations and Clinical Applications: A Nursing Approach. Elsevier, 2015.

17 Eckelkamp, Stephanie. "The Surprising Reason You Shouldn't Chug Water with Your Meals." Prevention Magazine, Hearst Magazine Media, 18 Feb. 2016; Stoddard, Grant. "3 Slow Your Roll and Chew Your Food." Vice Health, Vice Media, 17 Dec. 2018.

18 Kaplan, Karen. "Experts Measure Food Waste Not in Dollars or Tons, but by Calories, Vitamins and Minerals." Los Angeles Times, Los Angeles Times, 17 May 2017.

19 Kaplan. "Experts Measure Food Waste Not in Dollars or Tons, but by Calories, Vitamins and Minerals." Los Angeles Times, 2017.

20 Hanson, Craig, et al. "What's Food Loss and Waste Got to Do with Climate Change? A Lot, Actually." World Resources Institute, World Resources Institute, 26 Sept. 2018.

21 Hanson, et al. "What's Food Loss and Waste Got to Do with Climate Change? A Lot, Actually." 2018.

22 Hanson, et al., 2018.

23 Hamblin, James. "Science Compared Every Diet, and the Winner Is Real Food." The Atlantic, Atlantic Media Company, 24 Mar. 2014.

24 Rutledge, Kim, et al. "Omnivore." National Geographic Resource Library, National Geographic Society, 21 Jan. 2011; Hamblin, James. "Science Compared Every Diet, and the Winner Is Real Food." The Atlantic, Atlantic Media Company, 24 Mar. 2014.

25 Manzel, Arndt, et al. "Role of 'Western Diet' in Inflammatory Autoimmune Diseases." Current Allergy and Asthma Reports, U.S. National Library of Medicine, Jan. 2014.

26 Manzel, et al. "Role of 'Western Diet' in Inflammatory Autoimmune Diseases." 2014.

27 McManus, Katherine D. "What Is a Plant-Based Diet and Why Should You Try It?" Harvard Medical School, Harvard Health Publishing, 27 Sept. 2018.

28 Battaglia Richi, Evelyne, et al. "Health Risks Associated with Meat Consumption: A Review of Epidemiological Studies." International Journal for Vitamin and Nutrition Research, U.S. National Library of Medicine, 2015; Sandoiu, Ana. "The Effects of Antibiotic Use in Animals on Human Health and the Drug Resistance Crisis." Medical News Today, MediLexicon International, 9 Nov. 2018; Rouhani, Mohammad, et al. "- Is there a relationship between red or processed meat intake and obesity? A systematic review and meta-analysis of observational studies." Obesity Reviews 15 (9), 2014.

29 Eng, Monica. "The Costs of Cheap Meat." Chicago Tribune, Chicago Tribune, 24 Sept. 2010.

30 Jones, Keithly, et al. "Per Capita Red Meat and Poultry Disappearance: Insights into Its Steady Growth." USDA Economic Research Service, United States Department of Agriculture, 4 June 2018.

31 Hyman, Mark. "Why I Am a Pegan – or Paleo-Vegan – and Why You Should Be Too!" Dr. Mark Hyman, Mark Hyman, 7 Nov. 2014.

32 Spritzler, Franziska. "21 Reasons to Eat Real Food." Healthline, Healthline Media, 12 Apr. 2019.

33 Gunnars, Kris. "Processed Foods: Health Risks and Dangers." Medical News Today, MediLexicon International, 1 Aug. 2017.

34 Spritzler, Franziska. "21 Reasons to Eat Real Food." Healthline, Healthline Media, 12 Apr. 2019.

35 Gunnars. "Processed Foods: Health Risks and Dangers." 2017.

36 Gunnars, 2017.

37 Bell, Victoria, et al. "One Health, Fermented Foods, and Gut Microbiota." Foods (Basel, Switzerland), MDPI, 3 Dec. 2018.

38 Bell, "One Health, Fermented Foods, and Gut Microbiota." 2018.

39 Center for Food Safety and Applied Nutrition. "Guidance on Developing and Using Data Bases for Nutrition Labeling." 2018.

40 Center for Food Safety and Applied Nutrition. "Guidance on Developing and Using Data Bases for Nutrition Labeling." U.S. Food and Drug Administration, FDA, 20 Jan. 2018.

41 Alcock, Joe, et al. "Is Eating Behavior Manipulated by the Gastrointestinal Microbiota? Evolutionary Pressures and Potential Mechanisms." BioEssays : News and Reviews in Molecular, Cellular and Developmental Biology, WILEY Periodicals, Inc., Oct. 2014.

42 Jabr, Ferris. "How Sugar and Fat Trick the Brain into Wanting More Food." Scientific American, Scientific American, 1 Jan. 2016.

43 Harvard Health Publishing. "The Sweet Danger of Sugar." Harvard Medical School, Harvard Health Publishing, 5 Nov. 2019.

44 Morris, Michael J, et al. "Salt Craving: The Psychobiology of Pathogenic Sodium Intake." Physiology & Behavior, U.S. National Library of Medicine, 6 Aug. 2008.

45 "The Sweet Danger of Sugar." Harvard Medical School, Harvard Health Publishing, 5 Nov. 2019.

46 Gunnars, Kris. "Types of Salt: Himalayan vs Kosher vs Regular vs Sea Salt." Healthline, Healthline Media, 19 Oct. 2018; Group, Edward. "The Health Dangers of Table Salt." Global Healing Center, Global Healing Center, 24 Jan. 2017.

47 Caporuscio, Jessica. "Sea Salt vs. Table Salt: Differences and Health Benefits." Medical News Today, MediLexicon International, 1 Oct. 2019.

48 Fuhrman, Joel. "The Hidden Dangers of Fast and Processed Food." American Journal of Lifestyle Medicine, SAGE Publications, 3 Apr. 2018.

49 Price, Annie. "Is Pink Himalayan Salt Any Better Than Table Salt?" Dr. Axe, Dr. Axe, 19 Aug. 2019.

50 Price. "Is Pink Himalayan Salt Any Better Than Table Salt?" Dr. Axe, 2019.

51 Darcey, Melissa. "How Your Body Extracts Nutrients from Food, Part 2." Pathway Genomics, Pathway Genomics, 3 Apr. 2018.

52 Eckelkamp, Stephanie. "The Surprising Reason You Shouldn't Chug Water with Your Meals." Prevention Magazine, Hearst Magazine Media, 18 Feb. 2016.

53 Brodwin, Erin. "There's Even More Evidence That One Type of Diet Is the Best for Your Body and Brain." Business Insider, Insider Inc., 2 Jan. 2019.

54 Zmora, N., Suez, J. & Elinav, E. "You are what you eat: diet, health and the gut microbiota." Nat Rev Gastroenterol Hepatol (16), 2019.

55 Conlon, Michael A, and Anthony R Bird. "The Impact of Diet and Lifestyle on Gut Microbiota and Human Health." Nutrients, MDPI, 24 Dec. 2014.

56 Manzel, Arndt, et al. "Role of 'Western Diet' in Inflammatory Autoimmune Diseases." Current Allergy and Asthma Reports, U.S. National Library of Medicine, Jan. 2014.

57 Zinöcker, Marit K, and Inge A Lindseth. "The Western Diet-Microbiome-Host Interaction and Its Role in Metabolic Disease." Nutrients, MDPI, 17 Mar. 2018; Moss, Michael. "The Extraordinary Science of Addictive Junk Food." The New York Times, The New York Times, 20 Feb. 2013.

58 Cassetty, Samantha. "What Is Healthier: Natural Sugar, Table Sugar or Artificial Sweeteners?" NBCNews.com, NBCUniversal News Group, 6 Apr. 2018.

59 Villines, Zawn. "Is Sugar in Fruit Bad for You?" Medical News Today, MediLexicon International, 25 June 2019; Dennett, Carrie. "The Sugar in Fruit Doesn't Make It Bad for You, despite Some Trendy Diet Claims." The Washington Post, WP Company, 16 Apr. 2019.

60 "Carbohydrates and Blood Sugar." The Nutrition Source, Harvard T. H. Chan School of Public Health, 25 July 2016.

61 "Added Sugars." American Heart Association, American Heart Association, Inc., 17 Apr. 2018.

62 Jabr, Ferris. "How Sugar and Fat Trick the Brain into Wanting More Food." Scientific American, Scientific American, 1 Jan. 2016.

63 Moss, Michael. "The Extraordinary Science of Addictive Junk Food." The New York Times, The New York Times, 20 Feb. 2013.

64 Malito, Alessandra. "Grocery Stores Carry 40,000 More Items than They Did in the 1990s." MarketWatch, MarketWatch, Inc., 17 June 2017.

65 Katch, Victor. "Fake Food." Michigan Today, The Regents of the University of Michigan, 6 Mar. 2017.

66 Katch. "Fake Food." The Regents of the University of Michigan, 2017.

67 Astrup, Arne, and Susanne Bügel. "Overfed but Undernourished: Recognizing Nutritional Inadequacies/Deficiencies in Patients with Overweight or Obesity." International Journal of Obesity, U.S. National Library of Medicine, 6 July 2018.

68 MacDonald, Ann. "Why Eating Slowly May Help You Feel Full Faster." Harvard Medical School, Harvard Health Publishing, 19 Oct. 2010.

69 Milanowski, Ann. "Don't Eat Until You're Full – Instead, Mind Your Hara Hachi Bu Point." Health Essentials from Cleveland Clinic, Cleveland Clinic, 4 June 2019.

70 Greer, Stephanie M, et al. "The Impact of Sleep Deprivation on Food Desire in the Human Brain." Nature Communications, U.S. National Library of Medicine, 2013.

71 Kilburn, Marianna. "5 Foods You Might Crave If You're Sleep Deprived." A.Vogel Herbal Remedies, A. Vogel , 12 Dec. 2018.

72 Gazan, Rozenn, et al. "Drinking Water Intake Is Associated with Higher Diet Quality among French Adults." Nutrients, MDPI, 31 Oct. 2016.

73 Fuhrman, Joel, et al. "Changing Perceptions of Hunger on a High Nutrient Density Diet." Nutrition Journal, BioMed Central, 7 Nov. 2010.

74 LeWine, Howard. "Distracted eating may lead to weight gain." Harvard Medical School, Harvard Health Publishing, 29 Mar. 2013; "Mindful eating." Harvard Medical School, Harvard Health Publishing, Feb. 2011.

75 Gannon, Mary Carol, and Frank Quentin Nuttall. "Effect of a High-Protein Diet on Ghrelin, Growth Hormone, and Insulin-like Growth Factor-I and Binding Proteins 1 and 3 in Subjects with Type 2 Diabetes Mellitus." Metabolism: Clinical and Experimental, U.S. National Library of Medicine, Sept. 2011.

76 Harvard Health Publishing. "Protect Your Brain With 'Good' Fat." Harvard Medical School, Harvard Health Publishing, Sept. 2012.; "Weight Loss: Feel Full on Fewer Calories." Mayo Clinic, Mayo Foundation for Medical Education and Research, 20 Jan. 2017.

77 Aswell, Sarah. "Fiber Diet: How It Changes Your Gut and How to Eat More." Healthline, Healthline Media, 17 Sept. 2018.

78 Theobald, Mikel. "7 Hypothyroidism-Friendly Foods to Add to Your Diet." Everyday Health, Everyday Health, Inc., 25 Feb. 2019.

79 Katz, Rebecca. The Longevity Kitchen: Satisfying, Big-Flavor Recipes Featuring the Top 16 Age-Busting Power Foods. Ten Speed Press, 2013.

80 Katz, The Longevity Kitchen: Satisfying, Big-Flavor Recipes Featuring the Top 16 Age-Busting Power Foods. 2013.

81 Ware, Megan. "Green Tea: Health Benefits, Side Effects, and Research." Medical News Today, MediLexicon International, 28 Mar. 2017.

82 Wang, Hu, et al. "Plants vs. Cancer: A Review on Natural Phytochemicals in Preventing and Treating Cancers and Their Druggability." Anti-Cancer Agents in Medicinal Chemistry, U.S. National Library of Medicine, Dec. 2012.

83 Arnarson, Atli. "Walnuts 101: Nutrition Facts and Health Benefits." Healthline, Healthline Media, 26 Mar. 2019.

84 Posch, Linda. "Health Benefits of Walnut Oil." What's Cooking America, What's Cooking America, 7 Oct. 2016.

85 Posch, "Health Benefits of Walnut Oil." 2016.

86 Axe, Josh. "Top 10 Benefits of Flaxseed and How to Add Them to Your Diet." Dr. Axe, Dr. Axe, 25 Jun. 2019.

87 Zeratsky, Katherine. "Does Ground Flaxseed Have More Health Benefits Than Whole Flaxseed?" The Mayo Clinic, Mayo Foundation for Medical Education and Research, 18 Jan. 2019.

88 Favret, Jenny. "Water Is the Healthiest Option." Duke Health Blog, Duke Health, 1 July 2015.

89 Gazan, Rozenn, et al. "Drinking Water Intake Is Associated with Higher Diet Quality among French Adults." Nutrients, MDPI, 31 Oct. 2016.

90 Popkin, Barry M, et al. "Water, Hydration, and Health." Nutrition Reviews, U.S. National Library of Medicine, Aug. 2010.

91 Nagdeve, Meenakshi, and Ishani Bose. "8 Amazing Hibiscus Tea Health Benefits." Organic Facts, Organic Information Services, 23 Jan. 2020.

92 Nagdeve, et al. "8 Amazing Hibiscus Tea Health Benefits." 2020.

93 McManus, Katherine D. "What Is a Plant-Based Diet and Why Should You Try It?" Harvard Medical School, Harvard Health Publishing, 27 Sept. 2018.

94 The US Burden of Disease Collaborators. "The State of US Health, 1990-2016: Burden of Diseases, Injuries, and Risk Factors Among US States." JAMA 319(14), American Medical Association, 2018.

95 Anaïs, Rico-Campà, et al. "Association between consumption of ultra-processed foods and all-cause mortality: SUN prospective cohort study." BMJ (365), The BMJ Publishing Group, 2019.

96 Springmann, M., et al. "Options for keeping the food system within environmental limits." Nature (562), 2018.

FOOD IS MEDICINE

97 Sender, Ron, et al. "Revised Estimates for the Number of Human and Bacteria Cells in the Body." PLoS Biology, Public Library of Science, 19 Aug. 2016; Maynard, Amanda. ACLS Training Center, ACLS Training Center, https://www.acls.net/study-guide-body-systems.htm.

98 Fletcher, Jenna. "6 Essential Nutrients: Sources and Why You Need Them." Medical News Today, Healthline Media UK, 22 Aug. 2019.

99 "What Is a Gene?" U.S. National Library of Medicine, National Institutes of Health, 10 Dec. 2019.

100 Kirkpatrick, Bailey. "Epigenetics, Nutrition, and Our Health: How What We Eat Could Affect Tags on Our DNA." What Is Epigenetics?, What Is Epigenetics?, 15 May 2018.

101 Kirkpatrick, "Epigenetics, Nutrition, and Our Health...", 2018.

102 Katherine Zeratsky, R.D. "What Are Functional Foods?" Mayo Clinic, Mayo Foundation for Medical Education and Research, 21 Feb. 2018.

103 Klemm, Sarah. "Functional Foods." EatRight, Academy of Nutrition and Dietetics, 15 July 2019.

104 "Feed Your Genes: How Our Genes Respond to the Foods We Eat." ScienceDaily, ScienceDaily and The Norwegian University of Science and Technology, 20 Sept. 2011.

105 "Nutrition and Health Are Closely Related." Health.Gov, Office of Disease Prevention and Health Promotion, 26 Aug. 2015.

106 Murray, Michael T., et al. The Encyclopedia of Healing Foods. Atria Books, 2010.

107 Murray, et al. The Encyclopedia of Healing Foods, 2010.

108 Murray, et al. The Encyclopedia of Healing Foods, 2010.

109 Murray, et al. The Encyclopedia of Healing Foods, 2010.

110 "1/3 Cup Whole Almonds." FatSecret with information from USDA, FatSecret, 4 Feb. 2008.

111 Murray, et al. The Encyclopedia of Healing Foods, 2010.

112 Brazier, Yvette. "Almonds: Health Benefits, Nutrition, and Risks." Medical News Today, H, 12 Dec. 2019.

113 Leech, Joe. "9 Evidence-Based Health Benefits of Almonds." Healthline, Healthline Media, 12 Dec. 2019.

114 Benediktsdottir, Audur. "Raw vs Roasted Nuts: Which Is Healthier?" Healthline, Healthline Media, 19 Aug. 2017.

115 Murray, et al. The Encyclopedia of Healing Foods, 2010.

116 Murray, et al. The Encyclopedia of Healing Foods, 2010.

117 Kuddus, Mohammed. Enzymes in Food Biotechnology: Production, Applications, and Future Prospects. Academic Press, an Imprint of Elsevier, 2019.

118 Lee, Matthew. "Which Amino Acids Are in Grains?" SF Gate, Hearst Newspapers, 17 Dec. 2018.

119 "Is Amaranth Gluten-free?" Beyond Celiac, Beyond Celiac.

120 Chmelik, Zdeněk, et al. "Amaranth as a Potential Dietary Adjunct of Lifestyle Modification to Improve Cardiovascular Risk Profile." Science Direct: Nutrition Research, Elsevier, 22 Oct. 2019.

121 Murray, et al. The Encyclopedia of Healing Foods, 2010; Huang, et al. "The Role of Selenium in Inflammation and Immunity: from Molecular Mechanisms to Therapeutic Opportunities." 2012.

122 Mandl, Elise. "7 Proven Health Benefits of Brazil Nuts." Healthline, Healthline Media, 7 May 2019.

123 Huang, et al. "The Role of Selenium in Inflammation and Immunity: from Molecular Mechanisms to Therapeutic Opportunities." 2012.

124 "Chromium in the Diet." EUFIC, European Food Information Council, 27 Mar. 2019.

125 Romero, Melissa. "The Powerful Health Benefits of Buckwheat: Washingtonian (DC)." Washingtonian, Washingtonian Media Inc., 8 May 2012.

126 Arnarson, Atli. "Buckwheat 101: Nutrition Facts and Health Benefits." Healthline, Healthline Media, 10 May 2019.

127 Arnarson, "Buckwheat 101...", 2019.

128 Arnarson, "Buckwheat 101...", 2019.

129 Arnarson, "Buckwheat 101...", 2019.

130 McDermott, Annette. "Carob Powder: 9 Nutrition Facts and Health Benefits." Healthline, Healthline Media, 28 Nov. 2016.

131 Papaefstathiou, Eleni, et al. "Nutritional Characterization of Carobs and Traditional Carob Products." Food Science & Nutrition, John Wiley and Sons Inc., 4 Oct. 2018.

132 Murray, et al. The Encyclopedia of Healing Foods, 2010.

133 "Cashews." The World's Healthiest Foods, The George Mateljan Foundation.

134 Soares, Denise Josino, et al. "Prevalent Fatty Acids in Cashew Nuts Obtained from Conventional and Organic Cultivation in Different Stages of Processing." Food Science and Technology, Campinas, 33(2), Apr-Jun. 2013.

135 "Cashews." The World's Healthiest Foods, The George Mateljan Foundation.

136 "Chia Seed History and Origin." Ancient Grains, 20 Mar. 2015.

137 "Seeds, Chia Seeds, Dried Nutrition Facts & Calories." Self: Nutrition Data, Condé Nast, from USDA.

138 Gunnars, Kris. "11 Proven Health Benefits of Chia Seeds." Healthline, Healthline Media, 8 Aug. 2018

139 Murray, et al. The Encyclopedia of Healing Foods, 2010.

140 "Chickpeas (Garbanzo Beans)." Harvard T.H. Chan School of Public Health, Harvard University, 28 Oct. 2019.

141 Elliott, Brianna. "8 Health and Nutrition Benefits of Chickpeas." Healthline, Healthline Media, 7 May 2018.

142 Tannis, Allison. Feed Your Skin, Starve Your Wrinkles: Eat Your Way to Firmer, More Beautiful Skin With the 100 Best Anti-Aging Foods. Fair Winds Press, 2009.

143 Vally, Hassan, and Neil LA Misso. "Adverse reactions to the sulphite additives." Gastroenterology and hepatology from bed to bench vol. 5,1, 2012.

144 Murray, et al. The Encyclopedia of Healing Foods, 2010.

145 Leonard, Jayne. "Monolaurin: Benefits, Uses, Forms, and Side Effects." Medical News Today, Healthline Media UK, 2 Oct. 2017.

146 "Nuts, Coconut Meat, Raw." U.S. Department of Agriculture, U.S. Department of Agriculture, 1 Apr. 2019.; "Manganese: Fact Sheet for Health Professionals." NIH: Office of Dietary Supplements, U.S. Department of Health and Human Services, 6 Sept. 2019.;

147 Murray, et al. The Encyclopedia of Healing Foods, 2010; Axe, Josh. "Coconut Oil Benefits, Nutrition and Popular Uses." Dr. Axe, Dr. Axe, 24 Apr. 2019.

148 Ramsden, Christopher E, et al. "Re-evaluation of the traditional diet-heart hypothesis: analysis of recovered data from Minnesota Coronary Experiment (1968-73)." BMJ, BMJ Publishing Group, 2016.

149 Mahdy Ali, K, et al. "Cardiovascular Disease Risk Reduction by Raising HDL Cholesterol--Current Therapies and Future Opportunities." British Journal of Pharmacology, Blackwell Publishing Ltd, Nov. 2012; Cardoso, Diuli A, et al. "A Coconut Extra Virgin Oil-Rich Diet Increases HDL Cholesterol and Decreases Waist Circumference and Body Mass in Coronary Heart Disease Patients." Nutricion Hospitalaria, U.S. National Library of Medicine, 1 Nov. 2015

150 Wang, Baogui, et al. "Effects of Long-Chain and Medium-Chain Fatty Acids on Apoptosis and Oxidative Stress in Human Liver Cells with Steato-

sis." Journal of Food Science, U.S. National Library of Medicine, Mar. 2016.

151 Murray, Michael T., et al. The Encyclopedia of Healing Foods. Atria Books, 2010.

152 Bjarnadottir, Adda. "Flax Seeds 101: Nutrition Facts and Health Benefits." Healthline, Healthline Media, 28 Mar. 2019.

153 Bjarnadottir, "Flax Seeds 101...", 2019.

154 Bjarnadottir, "Flax Seeds 101...", 2019.

155 "Omega-3 Fatty Acids: Fact Sheet for Health Professionals." NIH Office of Dietary Supplements, U.S. Department of Health and Human Services, 17 Oct. 2019.

156 Bjarnadottir, "Flax Seeds 101...", 2019.

157 Bjarnadottir, "Flax Seeds 101...", 2019.

158 Ruggeri, Christine. "Hemp Seeds Benefits for Pain, Weight Loss and More." Dr. Axe, Dr. Axe, 22 Sept. 2019.

159 Crichton-Stuart, Cathleen. "9 Benefits of Hemp Seeds: Nutrition, Health, and Use." Medical News Today, Healthline Media UK, 11 Sept. 2018.

160 Crichton-Stuart, "9 Benefits of Hemp Seeds: Nutrition, Health, and Use." 2018.

161 Crichton-Stuart, "9 Benefits of Hemp Seeds: Nutrition, Health, and Use." 2018.

162 Pearson, Keith. "Is Pink Himalayan Salt Better Than Regular Salt?" Healthline, Healthline Media, 16 May 2017.

163 Pearson. "Is Pink Himalayan Salt Better Than Regular Salt?" 2017.

164 Pearson. "Is Pink Himalayan Salt Better Than Regular Salt?" 2017.

165 Pearson. "Is Pink Himalayan Salt Better Than Regular Salt?" 2017.

166 Buettner, Kristin. "Kelp Benefits: Boost Your Health with Seaweed." Healthline, Healthline Media, 11 Oct. 2017.

167 Moussavou, Ghislain, et al. "Anticancer Effects of Different Seaweeds on Human Colon and Breast Cancers." MDPI: Marine Drugs, National Center for Biotechnology Information, 24 Sept. 2014.

168 Choudhry, Hani, et al. "Iodine Consumption and Cognitive Performance: Confirmation of Adequate Consumption." Food Science & Nutrition, National Center for Biotechnology Information, 1 June 2018.

169 Nagdeve, Meenakshi. "Seaweed Health Benefits, Nutrition, Uses & Side Effects." Organic Facts, Organic Information Services, 20 Dec. 2019.

170 Nagdeve. "Seaweed Health Benefits, Nutrition, Uses & Side Effects." 2019.

171 O'Hara, Julie. "Lentils: A Legume for The Ages." NPR, NPR, 7 Jan. 2009.

172 "Lentils Significantly Reduce Blood Glucose Levels." ScienceDaily, ScienceDaily, 13 June 2018.

173 Adebamowo, Clement A., et al. "Dietary Flavanols and Flavanol-Rich Foods Intake and the Risk of Breast Cancer." Wiley Online Library, International Journal of Cancer, 8 Feb. 2005.

174 Murray, Michael T., et al. The Encyclopedia of Healing Foods. Atria Books, 2010.

175 "Millet, Raw Nutrition Facts & Calories." Self: Nutrition Data, Condé Nast, from USDA.

176 "Food Sensitivities." The World's Healthiest Foods, The George Mateljan Foundation.

177 High Fiber, Whole Grains Linked to Lower CVD, Diabetes, Cancer Risk." Medscape, WebMD, LLC, 15 Jan. 2019.

178 Murray, Michael T, et al. The Encyclopedia of Healing Foods, 2010.

179 "Miso: Nutrition and Health Benefits." Berkeley Wellness, Remedy Health Media, 12 Oct. 2016; "Miso Nutrition Facts & Calories." Self: Nutrition Data, Condé Nast, from USDA.

180 "Miso: Nutrition and Health Benefits." 2016.

181 Dresden, Danielle. "Top 5 Nutritional Yeast Benefits and How to Use It." Medical News Today, Healthline Media UK, 3 Oct. 2018.

182 Julson, Erica. "Why Is Nutritional Yeast Good for You?" Healthline, Healthline Media, 30 Nov. 2017.

183 Julson. "Why Is Nutritional Yeast Good for You?" 2017.

184 Julson. "Why Is Nutritional Yeast Good for You?" 2017.

185 Murray, Michael T, et al. The Encyclopedia of Healing Foods, 2010.

186 Bjarnadottir, Adda. "Oats 101: Nutrition Facts and Healh Benefits." Healthline, Healthline Media, 17 May 2019.

187 "Oats." The Nutrition Source, Harvard T.H. Chan School of Public Health, 4 Nov. 2019.

188 Zeratsky, Katherine. "Why Choose Olive Oil over Other Fats?" Mayo Clinic, Mayo Foundation for Medical Education and Research, 25 Oct. 2019.

189 Guasch-Ferré, Marta, et al. "Olive Oil Intake and Risk of Cardiovascular Disease and Mortality in the PREDIMED Study." BMC Medicine, National Center for Biotechnology Medicine, 13 May 2014.

190 Leech, Joe. "11 Proven Benefits of Olive Oil." Healthline, Healthline Media, 14 Sep. 2018.

191 Leech. "11 Proven Benefits of Olive Oil." 2018.

192 Murray, Michael T, et al. The Encyclopedia of Healing Foods, 2010.

193 "Nuts, Pine Nuts, Dried Nutrition Facts & Calories." Self: Nutrition Data, Condé Nast, from USDA. (from USDA)

194 Harvard Health Publishing. "Vitamins and Your Heart." Harvard Health, Harvard Medical School; Tremblay, Sylvie. "Vitamins & Minerals That Affect the Heart." Healthy Eating | SF Gate, Hearst Newspapers, 6 Dec. 2018.

195 Murray, Michael T., et al. The Encyclopedia of Healing Foods, 2010.

196 "Nuts, Pistachio Nuts, Dry Roasted, without Salt Added Nutrition Facts & Calories." Self: Nutrition Data, Condé Nast, from USDA.

197 West, Sheila G, et al. "Diets Containing Pistachios Reduce Systolic Blood Pressure and Peripheral Vascular Responses to Stress in Adults with Dyslipidemia." Hypertension, National Center for Biotechnology Information, July 2012.

198 Paterniti, Irene, et al. "The Anti-Inflammatory and Antioxidant Potential of Pistachios (Pistacia Vera L.) In Vitro and In Vivo." MDPI Nutrients, National Center for Biotechnology Information, 22 Aug. 2017.

199 McDermott, Annette. "Can Pumpkin Seeds Improve My Prostate Health?" Healthline, Healthline Media, 6 Jul. 2016.

200 Shubrook, Nicola, and Kerry Torrens. "The Health Benefits of Pumpkin Seeds." BBC Good Food, Immediate Media Company Limited, 1 Oct. 2018.

201 Murray, Michael T. The Encyclopedia of Healing Foods, 2010.

202 Ware, Megan, "Quinoa: Nutrition, Health Benefits, and Dietary Tips." Medical New Today, Healthline Media UK, 15 Nov. 2019.

203 Murray, Michael T, et al. The Encyclopedia of Healing Foods, 2010.

204 Kandola, Aaron. "Simple Carbs vs. Complex Carbs: What's the Difference?" Medical News Today, Healthline Media UK, 14 May 2019.

205 Murray, Michael T., et al. The Encyclopedia of Healing Foods. Atria Books, 2010.

206 Leech, Joe. "10 Health Benefits of Spirulina." Healthline, Healthline Media, 5 Oct. 2018.

207 Leech, Joe. "10 Health Benefits of Spirulina." Healthline, Healthline Media, 5 Oct. 2018.

208 Lall, U.B. Journey to a Healthy Life. Notion Press, 22 May 2019.

209 Lall. Journey to Healthy Life. 2019.

210 Murray, Michael T., et al. The Encyclopedia of Healing Foods. Atria Books, 2010.

211 Murray, et al. The Encyclopedia of Healing Foods. 2010.

212 Corliss, Julie. "Folic Acid, a B Vitamin, Lowers Stroke Risk in People with High Blood Pressure." Harvard Health Blog, Harvard Health Publishing, 29 Nov. 2016.

213 Huang, Zhi, et al. "The Role of Selenium in Inflammation and Immunity: from Molecular Mechanisms to Therapeutic Opportunities." Antioxidants & Redox Signaling, Mary Ann Liebert, Inc., 1 Apr. 2012.

214 "Sesame Seeds Properties." Botanical Online, Botanical Online, 22 Apr. 2019

215 "Sesame Seeds Properties." 2019; Borenstein, Amy R., and James A. Mortimer. Alzheimers Disease: Life Course Perspectives on Risk Reduction. Elsevier/AP, Academic Press Is an Imprint of Elsevier, 2016; 3 Vitamins That Are Best for Boosting Your Immunity." Health Essentials from Cleveland Clinic, Cleveland Clinic, 2 Jan. 2020.

216 "Information about the Musculoskeletal and Skin Systems." NIH Curriculum Supplement Series, U.S. National Library of Medicine, 2007.

217 Ware, Megan. "Tahini: Nutrition, Benefits, Diet, and Risks." Medical News Today, Healthline Media UK, 23 Feb. 2018.

218 Murray, Michael T., et al. The Encyclopedia of Healing Foods, 2010.

219 "History." California Walnuts, California Walnut Board, 5 June 2019.

220 Ware, Megan. "Walnuts: Health Benefits, Nutrition, and Diet." Medical News Today, Healthline Media UK, 10 July 2018.

221 "Omega-3 Fatty Acids: Fact Sheet for Health Professionals." NIH Office of Dietary Supplements, U.S. Department of Health and Human Services, 17 Oct. 2019.

222 Arnarson, Atli. "Walnuts 101: Nutrition Facts and Health Benefits." Healthline, Healthline Media, 26 Mar. 2019.

223 Watanabe, Makoto, et al. "Identification of 6-Methylsulfinylhexyl Isothiocyanate as an Apoptosis-Inducing Component in Wasabi." Phytochemistry, U.S. National Library of Medicine, Mar. 2003.

224 Lu, Zhongjing, et al. "Antibacterial Activities of Wasabi against Escherichia Coli O157:H7 and Staphylococcus Aureus." Frontiers in Microbiology, US National Library of Medicine, 21 Sept. 2016.

225 Nagdeve, Meenakshi. "6 Wonderful Benefits of Wasabi." Organic Facts, Organic Information Services, 4 Oct. 2019.

226 Nagdeve. "6 Wonderful Benefits of Wasabi," 2019.

CULINARY PHARMACY

227 Opara., Elizabeth I., et al. "Culinary Herbs and Spices: Their Bioactive Properties, the Contribution of Polyphenols and the Challenges in Deducing Their True Health Benefits." MDPI, Multidisciplinary Digital Publishing Institute, 22 Oct. 2014

228 Mitscher, L.A. "Traditional Medicines." Comprehensive Medicinal Chemistry II, Elsevier, 11 Apr. 2007

229 Murray, Michael T., et al. The Encyclopedia of Natural Medicine, Third Edition. Atria Books, 2012.

230 Jiang, T. Alan. "Health Benefits of Culinary Herbs and Spices." Journal of AOAC International, U.S. National Library of Medicine, 1 Mar. 2019.

231 Vázquez-Fresno, Rosa, et al. "Herbs and Spices- Biomarkers of Intake Based on Human Intervention Studies – A Systematic Review." Genes & Nutrition, BioMed Central, 22 May 2019.

232 Jiang. "Health Benefits of Culinary Herbs and Spices." 2019.

233 Liao, Lian-Ying, et al. "A Preliminary Review of Studies on Adaptogens: Comparison of Their Bioactivity in TCM with That of Ginseng-like Herbs Used Worldwide." Chinese Medicine, BioMed Central, 16 Nov. 2018.

234 "WHO Global Report on Traditional and Complementary Medicine." World Health Organization, World Health Organization, 2019.

235 Wachtel-Galor S, Benzie IFF. Herbal Medicine: Biomolecular and Clinical Aspects. 2nd edition. CRC Press/Taylor & Francis, 2011.

236 Yee, Lisa M. Encyclopedia of Immigrant Health. Vol. 1, Springer, 2012.

237 Murray, Michael T., et al. The Encyclopedia of Healing Foods. Atria Books, 2010.

238 Link, Rachel. "7 Health Benefits and Uses of Anise Seed." Healthline, Healthline Media, 15 Oct. 2018.

239 Link. "7 Health Benefits." 2018.

240 Oliver, Kyra. "Bay Leaf Benefits for Digestion, Wounds and Diabetics." Dr. Axe, Dr. Axe. 3 Apr. 2017; Staughton, John. "Top 8 Benefits of Bay Leaves." Organic Facts, Organic Information Services, 19 Oct. 2019.

241 Staughton. "Top 8 Benefits of Bay Leaves." Organic Information Services, 19 Oct. 2019.

242 Staughton, John. "Top 8 Benefits of Bay Leaves," 2019.

243 Edwards, Rebekah. "Black Pepper Benefits, Uses, Nutrition and Recipes." Dr. Axe, Dr. Axe, 29 Apr. 2019.

244 Edwards. "Black Pepper Benefits, Uses, Nutrition and Recipes." 2019.

245 Edwards, 2019.

246 Katz. The Longevity Kitchen: Satisfying, Big-Flavor Recipes Featuring the Top 16 Age-Busting Power Foods. 2013; Murray, et al. The Encyclopedia of Healing Foods, 2010.

247 Sarvade, Dattatray, et al. "The Queen of Spices and Ayurveda: A Brief Review." International Journal of Research in Ayurveda and Pharmacy (7), 2016.

248 Nagdeve, Meenakshi, et al. "11 Evidence-Based Benefits of Cardamom." Organic Facts, Organic Information Services, 27 Jan. 2020.

249 Butt, Masood Sadiq, et al. "Anti-oncogenic Perspectives of Spices/Herbs: A Comprehensive Review." EXCLI Journal (12), National Center for Biotechnology Information. 17 Dec. 2013.

250 Kandikattu, Hemanth Kumar, et al. "Anti-Inflammatory and Anti-Oxidant Effects of Cardamom (Elettaria Repens (Sonn.) Baill) and Its Phytochemical Analysis by 4D GCXGC TOF-MS." Biomedicine & Pharmacotherapy, Elsevier Masson, July 2017; Nagdeve, Meenakshi, et al. "11 Evidence-Based Benefits of Cardamom." Organic Facts, Organic Information Services, 27 Jan. 2020.

251 Murray, et al. The Encyclopedia of Healing Foods, 2010.

252 Chauhan, Mukul. "Blood Circulation Stimulation Properties of Cayenne Pepper: A Review" ISOR Journal of Applied Chemistry (11), Research Gate, May 2018.

253 Murray, et al. The Encyclopedia of Healing Foods, 2010.; Zhang, Shiqi, et al. "Capsaicin Reduces Blood Glucose by Increasing Insulin Levels and Glycogen Content Better than Capsiate in Streptozotocin-Induced Diabetic Rats." Journal of Agricultural and Food Chemistry, U.S. National Library of Medicine, 22 Mar. 2017.

254 Ruggeri, Christine. "Cayenne Pepper Benefits, Nutrition, Uses and Recipes." Dr. Axe, 17 Sept. 2019.

255 Carlsen, Monica H, et al. "The Total Antioxidant Content of More than 3100 Foods, Beverages, Spices, Herbs and Supplements Used Worldwide." Nutrition Journal, BioMed Central, 22 Jan. 2010; Braun and Cohen, 2015.

256 Leech, Joe. "10 Evidence-Based Health Benefits of Cinnamon." Healthline, Healthline Media, 5 Jul. 2018.

257 Shishehbor, Farideh, et al. "Cinnamon Consumption Improves Clinical Symptoms and Inflammatory Markers in Women with Rheumatoid Arthritis." Journal of the American College of Nutrition, U.S. National Library of Medicine, 3 May 2018.

258 Braun, Lesley, and Marc Cohen. Herbs & Natural Supplements: An Evidence-Based Guide. Vol. 2, Elsevier Health Sciences, 2015.

259 Braun and Cohen. Herbs & Natural Supplements: An Evidence-Based Guide. 2015.

260 Leech. "10 Evidence-Based Health Benefits of Cinnamon." 2018.

261 Braun and Cohen. Herbs & Natural Supplements: An Evidence-Based Guide. 2015.

262 Braun and Cohen, 2015.

263 Nagdeve, Meenakshi, et al. "10 Amazing Benefits of Manganese." Organic Facts, Organic Information Services, 25 Dec. 2019.

264 Metropulos, Megan. "Cloves: Health Benefits and Uses." Medical News Today, Healthline Media UK, 30 Jan. 2018.

265 Metropulos. "Cloves: Health Benefits and Uses." 2018.

266 Murray, Michael T., et al. The Encyclopedia of Healing Foods. Atria Books, 2010; Katz. The Longevity Kitchen: Satisfying, Big-Flavor Recipes Featuring the Top 16 Age-Busting Power Foods. 2013; Streit, Lizzie. "10 Health Benefits of Cardamom, Backed by Science." Healthline, Healthline Media, 8 Aug. 2018.

267 Sharma, M.M., and R.K. Sharma. "Coriander." Handbook of Herbs and Spices (Second Edition), Woodhead Publishing, 27 Mar. 2014.

268 Nagdeve, Meenakshi. "12 Amazing Benefits of Cilantro or Coriander." Organic Facts, Organic Information Services, 26 Nov. 2019.

269 Harvard Health Publishing. "Can Everyday Spices Make You Healthier?" Harvard Medical School, Harvard Health Publishing, 19 Feb. 2016.

270 Olsen, Natalie. "Cumin Benefits." Healthline, Healthline Media, 8 Aug. 2017.

271 Amita, et al. "Cumin Seed Benefits, Usage, Side Effects – Ayurveda Details." Easy Ayurveda, Easy Ayurveda, 13 Nov. 2013.

272 Jadhav, Priyanka, et al. "Antiviral Potential of Selected Indian Medicinal (Ayurvedic) Plants against Herpes Simplex Virus 1 and 2." North American Journal of Medical Sciences, Medknow Publications & Media Pvt Ltd, Dec. 2012.

273 Ruggeri, Christine. "Cumin Seeds Help Digestion & Immune System." Dr. Axe, Dr. Axe, 27 Dec. 2018.

274 Ruggeri. "Cumin Seeds Help Digestion & Immune System." 2018.

275 Oliver, Kyla. "8 Surprising Dill Weed Benefits (#6 Is Energizing)." Dr. Axe, Dr. Axe, 3 Apr. 2016; Yili, A, et al. "Chemical composition of essential oil from seeds of Anethum graveolens cultivated in China." Springer Link, Chemistry of Natural Compounds (42), 2006.

276 Oliver. "8 Surprising Dill Weed Benefits (#6 Is Energizing)." Dr. Axe, Dr. Axe, 3 Apr. 2016.

277 Oliver. "8 Surprising Dill Weed Benefits (#6 Is Energizing)," 2016.

278 Nagdeve, Meenakshi, and Sakina Kheriwala. "Dill: How to Make & Health Benefits." Organic Facts, Organic Information Services, 5 Dec. 2019.

279 Murray, Michael T., et al. The Encyclopedia of Healing Foods. Atria Books, 2010; Jeffers, Laura. "6 Surprising Ways Garlic Boosts Your Health." Health Essentials from Cleveland Clinic, Cleveland Clinic, 19 Dec. 2018.

280 Axe, Josh. "7 Raw Garlic Benefits for Reversing Disease." Dr. Axe, Dr. Axe, 28 Aug. 2019.

281 Axe. "7 Raw Garlic Benefits for Reversing Disease." 2019.

282 Axe, "7 Raw Garlic Benefits..." 2019.

283 Axe, "7 Raw Garlic Benefits..." 2019.

284 Bayan, Leyla, et al. "Garlic: A Review of Potential Therapeutic Effects." Avicenna Journal of Phytomedicine, Mashhad University of Medical Sciences, Jan. 2014.

285 Braun and Cohen, 2015.

286 Bartels, E.M., et al. "Efficacy and Safety of Ginger in Osteoarthritis Patients: A Meta-Analysis of Randomized Placebo-Controlled Trials." Osteoarthritis and Cartilage, Volume 23, Science Direct, 7 Oct. 2014.

287 Braun and Cohen, 2015.

288 Cohen, Marc Maurice. "Tulsi - Ocimum Sanctum: An Herb for All Reasons." Journal of Ayurveda and Integrative Medicine, Medknow Publications & Media Pvt Ltd, 2014.

289 Levy, Jillian. "10 Holy Basil Benefits: Tulsi Helps Anxiety, Acne & More." Dr. Axe, Dr. Axe, 9 Jul. 2019.

290 Levy. "10 Holy Basil Benefits..." 2019.

291 Levy, 2019; Jaghsi, Sawsan, et al. "Relation Between Circulating Vitamin K1 and Osteoporosis in the Lumbar Spine in Syrian Post-Menopausal Women." The Open Rheumatology Journal, Bentham Open, 22 Jan. 2018.

292 Link, Rachel. "Horseradish Root Helps Prevent Respiratory Illness, UTIs & Cancer." Dr. Axe, Dr. Axe. 14 Aug. 2019.

293 Link. "Horseradish Root Helps Prevent Respiratory Illness, UTIs & Cancer." Dr. Axe. 14 Aug. 2019.

294 Link. "Horseradish Root Helps Prevent Respiratory Illness, UTIs & Cancer." 2019.

295 Link, Rachael. "How Leeks Can Protect You From Both Cancer & Heart Disease." Dr. Axe, Dr. Axe. 8 Sep. 2019; Kim, K.H., et al. "Antioxidant and Antimicrobial Activities of Ethanol Extract from Six Vegetables Containing Different Sulfur Compounds." Journal of the Korean Society of Food Science and Nutrition (41), 05 May 2012; Murray, Michael T., et al. The Encyclopedia of Healing Foods. Atria Books, 2010.

296 Petre, Alina. "10 Health and Nutrition Benefits of Leeks and Wild Ramps." Healthline, Healthline Media, 21 Jun. 2019; Poljšak, Borut, and Rok Fink. "The Protective Role of Antioxidants in the Defence against ROS/RNS-Mediated Environmental Pollution." Oxidative Medicine and Cellular Longevity, Hindawi Publishing Corporation, 2014.

297 Petre, Alina. "10 Health and Nutrition Benefits of Leeks and Wild Ramps." 2019.

298 "Folic Acid." Centers for Disease Control and Prevention, U.S. Department of Health and Human Services, 11 Apr. 2018.

299 Mercola, Joseph. "Lemongrass Oil Can Lighten Up Your Mood and More." Mercola, Dr. Joseph Mercola. 18 May 2017.

300 Naik, Morfan. "Antibacterial activity of lemongrass (Cymbopogon citratus) oil against some selected pathogenic bacterias." Asia Pacific Journal of Tropical Medicine, Elsevier, 20 Jul. 2010.

301 Katz, Rebecca. The Longevity Kitchen: Satisfying, Big-Flavor Recipes Featuring the Top 16 Age-Busting Power Foods. Ten Speed Press, 2013.

302 Nagdeve, Meenakshi. "13 Impressive Benefits of Mint Leaves." Organic Facts, Organic Information Services, 31 Dec. 2019.

303 Pearson, Keith. "8 Health Benefits of Mint." Healthline, Healthline Media, 13 Dec. 2017

304 Pearson. "8 Health Benefits of Mint." 2017.

305 "Manganese: Fact Sheet for Health Professionals." NIH: Office of Dietary Supplements, U.S. Department of Health and Human Services, 6 Sept. 2019.

306 Nagdeve, Meenakshi. "15 Impressive Uses & Benefits of Mustard." Organic Facts, Organic Information Services. 19 Oct. 2019.

307 Anisha, et al. "Sinigrin and Its Therapeutic Benefits." MDPI, Multidisciplinary Digital Publishing Institute, 29 Mar. 2016.

308 Castello, Marissa. "Ease Chest Congestion Naturally with a Mustard Pack" Dr. Marissa Castello, Dr. Marissa Castello, ND, 11 Jan. 2019.

309 Levy, Jillian. "Mustard Greens Nutrition, Health Benefits and Recipes." Dr. Axe, Dr. Axe, 24 Aug. 2019.

310 Katz, 2013.

311 Link. "Healthy Holiday Spice or Toxic Hallucinogen?" 2018.

312 Link, Rachael. "Healthy Holiday Spice or Toxic Hallucinogen?" Dr. Axe, Dr. Axe, 22 Dec. 2018

313 Katz, 2013; Ren, et al. "Evaluation of Polyphenolic Content and Antioxidant Activity in Two Onion Varieties Grown under Organic and Conventional Production Systems." 2017; Ahmed, et al. "Antibacterial Effect of Onion." Research Gate, Scholars Journal of Applied Medical Sciences (4), 30

Nov. 2016.

314 Kubala, Jillian. "9 Impressive Health Benefits of Onions." Healthline, Healthline Media. 18 Dec. 2018.

315 Kubala. "9 Impressive Health Benefits of Onions," 2018.

316 Ren, Feiyue, et al. "Evaluation of Polyphenolic Content and Antioxidant Activity in Two Onion Varieties Grown under Organic and Conventional Production Systems." Journal of the Science of Food and Agriculture, U.S. National Library of Medicine, July 2017.

317 Link, Rachel. "6 Science-Based Health Benefits of Oregano." Healthline, Healthline Media, 27 Oct. 2017.

318 Singletary, Keith. "Oregano: Overview of the Literature on Health Benefits." Research Gate, Nutrition Today (45), May 2010.

319 Katz, 2013.

320 Axe, Josh. "Oregano Oil Benefits for Infections, Fungus & Even the Common Cold." Dr. Axe, Dr. Axe, 26 Sept. 2018.

321 Axe. "Oregano Oil Benefits for Infections…" 2018.

322 Horne, Steven. "Oregano." The School of Modern Herbal Medicine, Tree of Light Publishing, 19 June 2013, modernherbalmedicine.com/articles/oregano.html.

323 Levy. "Parsley Benefits for Immunity, Digestion & More." 2019.

324 Murray, Michael T., et al. The Encyclopedia of Healing Foods. Atria Books, 2010.

325 Hill, Ansley. "7 Surprising Health Benefits of Parsley Root." Healthline, Healthline Media, 6 Jun. 2019; Ballatori, Nazzareno, et al. "Glutathione Dysregulation and the Etiology and Progression of Human Diseases." Biological Chemistry, U.S. National Library of Medicine, Mar. 2009.

326 Levy, Jillian. "Parsley Benefits for Immunity, Digestion & More." Dr. Axe, Dr. Axe. 12 Nov. 2019.

327 Marengo, Katherine. "5 Vitamins and Minerals to Boost Your Metabolism and Promote Weight Loss." Healthline, Healthline Media, 19 Dec. 2018.

328 Levy, Jillian. "Parsley Benefits for Immunity, Digestion & More." Dr. Axe, Dr. Axe. 12 Nov. 2019.; Link, Rachel "Surprising Benefits of Parsley Tea (And How to Make It)." Healthline, Healthline Media, 7 Mar. 2019.

329 Murray, et al. The Encyclopedia of Healing Foods. 2010.

330 Murray, et al. The Encyclopedia of Healing Foods. 2010.

331 Murray, et al. The Encyclopedia of Healing Foods, 2010. Braun and Cohen. Herbs & Natural Supplements: An Evidence-Based Guide. 2015.

332 Braun and Cohen, 2015.

333 Staughton, John. "16 Science-Backed Benefits of Rosemary." Organic Facts, Organic Information Services, 25 Nov. 2019.

334 Braun and Cohen, 2015.

335 Kamalipour, Maryam, and Shahin Akhondzadeh. "Cardiovascular Effects of Saffron: An Evidence-Based Review." The Journal of Tehran Heart Center, Tehran University of Medical Sciences, 2011; Abedimanesh, Nasim, et al. "Saffron and Crocin Improved Appetite, Dietary Intakes and Body Composition in Patients with Coronary Artery Disease." Journal of Cardiovascular and Thoracic Research, Tabriz University of Medical Sciences, 2017; Katz, Rebecca. The Longevity Kitchen: Satisfying, Big-Flavor Recipes Featuring the Top 16 Age-Busting Power Foods. Ten Speed Press, 2013.

336 Braun and Cohen, 2015.

337 Axe, Josh. "What is Sage Used For? Sage Benefits & Uses for Skin, Memory & More." Dr. Axe, Dr. Axe, 10 Apr. 2018.

338 Axe. "What Is Sage Used For?…" 2018.

339 Axe. "What Is Sage Used For?…" 2018.

340 Murray, et al. The Encyclopedia of Healing Foods. 2010.

341 Murray, et al, 2010.

342 Murray, et al, 2010.

343 Murray, et al, 2010.

344 Murray, et al, 2010.

345 Murray, et al, 2010.

346 Murray, et al, 2010.

347 Murray, et al, 2010.

348 Murray, et al, 2010.

349 Nickerson, Brittany Wood. Recipes from the Herbalist's Kitchen: Delicious, Nourishing Food for Lifelong Health and Well-Being. Storey Publishing, 2017; Enloe, Autumn. "8 Surprising Benefits and Uses of Tarragon." Healthline, Healthline Media, 11 Sept. 2018.

350 Price, Annie. "Thyme Benefits for Your Throat, Heart and Mood" Dr. Axe, Dr. Axe, 17 Jan. 2020; Vallverdú-Queralt, Anna, et al. "A Comprehensive Study on the Phenolic Profile of Widely Used Culinary Herbs and Spices: Rosemary, Thyme, Oregano, Cinnamon, Cumin and Bay." Food Chemistry, Elsevier, 8 Jan. 2014; Wang, Jingqiu, et al. "Antitumor, Antioxidant and Anti-Inflammatory Activities of Kaempferol and Its Corresponding Glycosides and the Enzymatic Preparation of Kaempferol." PLOS ONE, Public Library of Science, 17 May 2018.

351 Price, Annie. "Thyme Benefits for Your Throat, Heart and Mood" Dr. Axe, Dr. Axe, 17 Jan. 2020.

352 Price. "Thyme Benefits for Your Throat, Heart and Mood." 2020.

353 Price, 2020.

354 Braun and Cohen, 2015.

355 "Turmeric." National Center for Complementary and Integrative Health, U.S. Department of Health and Human Services, 27 Nov. 2018; Saini, Anu. "Physicians of Ancient India." Journal of Family Medicine and Primary Care 5 (2), 2016.

356 Braun and Cohen, 2015.

357 Braun and Cohen, 2015.

358 "Turmeric." National Center for Complementary and Integrative Health. 2018.

359 Wongcharoen, Wanwarang, et al. "Effects of Curcuminoids on Frequency of Acute Myocardial Infarction after Coronary Artery Bypass Grafting." The American Journal of Cardiology, U.S. National Library of Medicine, 1 July 2012.

CPSIA information can be obtained
at www.ICGtesting.com
Printed in the USA
JSHW071427160223
37833JS00003B/5

9 780996 432955